Lung Lifelines

Lung Lifelines

Nutrient-rich Melody Ensemble

Ehsan Sheroy

Spectra Enterprise

CONTENTS

Table of Content

Chapter 6: Spinach Serenity: Iron-rich Fuel for Respiration

6.1 Delve into the iron content of spinach and its impact on respiratory function

6.2 Easy-to-follow recipes that highlight spinach as a lung-friendly ingredient

6.3 Interviews with nutritionists and health experts emphasizing the link between iron and lung vitality

Chapter 7: Harmonizing Nutrients: The Complete Ensemble

7.1 Synthesize the nutritional elements discussed in previous chapters

7.2 Create comprehensive meal plans for lung health

7.3 Encourage readers to adopt a balanced, nutrient-rich lifestyle for sustained respiratory well-being

Introduction

In reality as we know it where the tune of prosperity is made out of the multifaceted transaction of wellbeing and nourishment, the ensemble of respiratory health stands apart as a critical refrain. The human lungs, similar to virtuoso instruments, assume a crucial part in the organization of life, supporting the musicality of breath that is frequently underestimated. Perceiving the significant association among sustenance and pneumonic essentialness, this investigation sets out on an excursion into the core of "Lung Helps: Supplement rich Tune Gathering."

At the center of this story lies an affirmation of the significance of lung wellbeing. Our respiratory framework, with its fragile and multifaceted construction, is defenseless to different difficulties that can think twice about capability. From contamination loaded air to the afflictions of current living, our lungs face a bunch of stressors that highlight the requirement for proactive consideration. It is inside this setting that the job of sustenance arises as a strong force to be reckoned with, equipped for blending the ensemble of respiratory prosperity.

The material whereupon this investigation unfurls is painted with the energetic tints of supplement rich food sources, each assuming an unmistakable part in strengthening the lungs. This excursion isn't simply a healthful aide yet an odyssey into understanding the powerful connection between what we consume and the versatility of our respiratory framework. The pages ahead wind around together the narratives of people whose lives have been moved by the extraordinary influence of supplement rich decisions, stressing the tune that unfurls when an ensemble of wellbeing is played couple with healthy nourishment.

As the suggestion unfurls, the main development presents the idea of pneumonic health. It illustrates the unpredictable dance between lung wellbeing and our decisions in our day to day routines. Here, the material is set, and the stage is enlightened for the nourishing ensemble that follows. The significance of understanding normal lung illnesses and their connections to consume less calories becomes evident, filling in as an impetus for the peruser to dive further into the story.

Moving consistently into the principal topical development, the spotlight falls on the little yet powerful blueberry. This supplement rich pearl becomes the overwhelming focus, uncovering its ability as a cell reinforcement force to be reckoned with. The section not just analyzes the logical underpinnings of blueberries' medical advantages yet additionally offers reasonable experiences into flawlessly integrating them into one's eating routine. Through stories and genuine tributes, the story takes on an individual touch, delineating the unmistakable effect that blueberries can have on respiratory prosperity.

As the orchestra advances, the rhythm movements to the omega-3 crescendo typified by salmon. This section plunges into the expanse of data encompassing omega-3 unsaturated fats and their significant mitigating properties. With a mix of culinary direction and healthful insight, perusers are directed through the consolidation of salmon into their dietary collection. The reverberation of salmon's dietary ensemble is reverberated in accounts of people who affect their lung wellbeing.

The kale development follows, revealing insight into this verdant green virtuoso and its rich nutrient substance. The part explains the job of kale in sustaining respiratory strength and presents imaginative ways of making it a staple in regular feasts. Grounded in logical comprehension and supplemented by down to earth exhortation, the kale development highlights the musical amicability attainable through careful wholesome decisions.

Turmeric becomes the dominant focal point in the ensuing development, offering a break of mitigating support for the lungs. The brilliant flavor, commended for its restorative properties, unfurls its true capacity as a culinary and helpful partner. Perusers are directed through the consolidation of turmeric into their feasts, opening the way to respiratory prosperity through a delightful and energizing excursion.

As the ensemble arrives at its penultimate development, the center movements to the iron-rich fuel of spinach. This part investigates the imperative job of iron in respiratory wellbeing and acquaints imaginative ways with imbue spinach into everyday cooking. Upheld by interviews with nutritionists and wellbeing specialists, the story highlights the cooperative connection between iron-rich sustenance and lung imperativeness.

The excellent finale gravitates toward with a thorough investigation of blending supplements, winding around together the different components introduced in before developments. This finishing up section integrates the dietary troupe, offering perusers a guide for making extensive dinner designs that focus on lung wellbeing. The finish of this musical excursion is a greeting for perusers to embrace an all encompassing and adjusted way to deal with nourishment, cultivating a long period of supported respiratory prosperity.

As the last notes of the orchestra disappear, the reverberation of Lung Life savers: Supplement rich Tune Troupe waits in the peruser's awareness, having a permanent impression of the perplexing association among sustenance and respiratory prosperity. The pages going before have spread out an embroidery of information, winding around together the narratives of supplement rich food varieties and the extraordinary effect they can have on the ensemble of lung wellbeing.

The excursion left upon isn't just a wholesome aide yet an odyssey into understanding the powerful connection between what we consume and the flexibility of our respiratory framework.

The material is painted with lively tints of blueberries, salmon, kale, turmeric, spinach, and a fitting troupe of supplements, each adding to the song of prosperity that reverberates through the pages.

At the core of this investigation lies the major acknowledgment of the meaning of lung wellbeing. In our current reality where the air we inhale is loaded down with poisons and the speed of life can be excited, our lungs stand as quiet sentinels, organizing the cadence of breath that supports life. The orchestra of respiratory health, as investigated in these sections, turns into a reference point, directing perusers toward a more profound enthusiasm for the imperative job nourishment plays in sustaining this fragile yet strong troupe of organs.

The suggestion, making way for this investigation, underlines the significance of understanding normal lung infirmities and their connections to slim down. It is a source of inspiration, welcoming perusers to play a functioning job in supporting their respiratory wellbeing through informed healthful decisions. The story unfurls naturally, similar as a melodic organization, where every part expands upon the former one, making a crescendo of information and motivation.

The principal development presents the idea of pneumonic wellbeing, offering an expansive point of view on the many-sided dance between way of life decisions and lung wellbeing. This central comprehension turns into the foundation whereupon the resulting developments are assembled. The orchestra picks up speed as the spotlight goes to blueberries, uncovering the cell reinforcement suggestion that this little yet strong organic product brings to the respiratory outfit.

The omega-3 crescendo follows, drove by the virtuoso salmon. As the story explores the tremendous expanse of data encompassing omega-3 unsaturated fats, perusers are directed through the reasonable parts of integrating salmon into their eating regimens. Genuine stories add an individual touch, outlining the significant effect that deliberate nourishing decisions can have on respiratory prosperity.

Kale becomes the overwhelming focus in the ensuing development, a verdant crescendo of nutrients sustaining respiratory strength. The part fills in as a healthful aide, offering down to earth guidance on flawlessly coordinating kale into everyday dinners. The ensemble turns into an embroidery of flavors and supplements, each adding to the amicable tune of lung wellbeing.

The interval is set apart by the brilliant flavor, turmeric, offering calming support for the lungs. The story unfurls the culinary and restorative capability of turmeric, welcoming perusers to appreciate its flavors while embracing its fortifying advantages. The ensemble turns into an excursion of revelation, where the wealth of flavors and supplements orchestrate to make a comprehensive way to deal with respiratory wellbeing.

The spinach development follows, a musical investigation of iron-rich fuel for breath. Through interviews with nutritionists and wellbeing specialists, the section clarifies the imperative job of iron in lung essentialness. The story turns into a discussion, connecting logical information with viable experiences, making the ensemble open to perusers of different foundations.

As the ensemble arrives at its penultimate development, the center movements to orchestrating supplements. This thorough investigation winds around together the different components introduced in before developments, making a union of information. Perusers are furnished with a guide for creating feast designs that focus on lung wellbeing, guaranteeing that the song of prosperity is supported in the cadence of day to day existence.

The excellent finale isn't simply an end yet a start — a solicitation to perusers to embrace an agreeable and adjusted way to deal with sustenance. The orchestra of Lung Life savers stretches out past the pages, resounding in the decisions in kitchens, supermarkets, and feasting tables. It turns into a long lasting excursion, where the song of respiratory health is supported through careful dietary decisions and a guarantee to generally prosperity.

In the finishing up notes, key focal points resonate — an update that the investigation is certainly not a transient second yet a supported obligation to lung wellbeing. The extra assets gave act as a compass, directing perusers on their continuous excursion of respiratory prosperity. As the last words wait on the page, the ensemble of Lung Helps keeps on repeating, motivating people to sustain their lungs and take in the completion of life's song.

Chapter 1

Prelude to Pulmonary Wellness

"Introduction to Pneumonic Wellbeing" unfurls as a thorough investigation of a progressive way to deal with respiratory wellbeing, winding around together the unpredictable embroidery of logical experiences, melodic treatment, and nourishing science. At the core of this creative drive lies the comprehension that all encompassing prosperity envelops the actual parts of wellbeing as well as the remedial force of workmanship and nourishment.

The excursion into this original worldview begins with a profound plunge into the domains of logical development. Pneumonic wellbeing, a basic feature of in general prosperity, has roused a committed group of specialists to dive into state of the art research. The interdisciplinary joint effort between pneumonic subject matter experts, specialists, and medical services experts frames the groundwork of Lung Life savers' spearheading drive. The preface makes way for an investigation into the unpredictable instruments of the respiratory framework, revealing insight into the significant ramifications of logical forward leaps for people looking to streamline their lung capability.

As the story unfurls, the spotlight goes to the extraordinary capability of melodic treatment in cultivating pneumonic health.

The Supplement rich Song Troupe, a focal part of Lung Helps' comprehensive methodology, is presented as a progressive combination of craftsmanship and science. Made by a group out of music specialists and achieved performers, the songs are not simple stylish articulations but rather remedial instruments finely tuned to synchronize with the cadenced examples of relaxing. This melodic orchestra draws in members in an agreeable dance of mending, encouraging respiratory strength through an exceptional type of pneumonic activity.

All the while, the preface stretches out its story strings to consolidate a nourishing aspect. Lung Life savers perceives that ideal respiratory wellbeing isn't exclusively reliant upon outside mediations yet is well established in the body's interior equilibrium. Teaming up with nutritionists, the drive presents an exceptionally formed dietary routine that fills in as a correlative power to the melodic treatment. Plentiful in fundamental nutrients and minerals known for their respiratory advantages, this wholesome part turns into a basic piece of the comprehensive structure, giving the body the sustenance essential for supporting ideal lung wellbeing.

A basic part of the preface is the acknowledgment that the Supplement rich Tune Outfit is intended for people across different socioeconomics. Respiratory prosperity is an all inclusive worry that rises above age, foundation, and wellbeing status. Whether one looks for preventive measures or addresses existing respiratory difficulties, the gathering offers a customized and versatile guide. The inclusivity of the program builds up its obligation to making pneumonic wellbeing open to a wide range of people, encouraging a culture of wellbeing that resounds with the different structure holding the system together.

Besides, Lung Helps positions the Supplement rich Song Group as in excess of a wellbeing program; it arises as a social power that broadens its impact into networks, schools, and medical services organizations. The preface features the drive's proactive commitment to local area effort and training. Studios, courses, and intuitive meetings become indispensable parts of the group's main goal, dispersing information and cultivating an aggregate comprehension of the complex association between respiratory wellbeing, music, and sustenance. Lung Life savers turns into an impetus for social change, moving a shift toward a respiratory prosperity ethos inside different networks.

The continuation of this account dives further into the logical underpinnings of the "Introduction to Aspiratory Wellbeing," disentangling the intricacies of respiratory wellbeing. As the material extends, the interdisciplinary coordinated effort between pneumonic subject matter experts, analysts, and medical care experts turns out to be more articulated. The conjunction of their skill blends into a rich embroidery of information that enlightens the complicated components overseeing the respiratory framework.

Inside the logical domain, an investigation of lung capability elements becomes basic. Pneumonic subject matter experts, furnished with cutting edge indicative devices and techniques, leave on an excursion to translate the nuanced interchange of aviation routes, alveoli, and bronchioles. This profound jump into the physical and physiological complexities of the respiratory framework clarifies the meaning of ideal lung capability in supporting generally wellbeing. The preface highlights the essential job of exploration in recognizing examples of respiratory misery, from normal illnesses to constant circumstances, accordingly preparing for designated mediations.

All the while, the story widens its degree to include the restorative domain of music. Music treatment, long recognized for its personal and mental advantages, becomes the dominant focal point as a creative methodology for advancing respiratory health. The Supplement rich Song Group, a demonstration of the combination of workmanship and science, is created with fastidious accuracy. The structures are custom-made for stylish satisfaction as well as with a restorative reason — to resound with the cadenced examples of relaxing. This collaboration makes a cooperative connection among music and respiratory capability, encouraging a climate where members can take part in a type of pneumonic activity that rises above the ordinary limits of customary treatments.

The preface additionally clarifies upon the mental components of the Supplement rich Song Outfit. Past its physiological advantages, the force of music to ease pressure, uneasiness, and mental exhaustion is stressed. As members drench themselves in the agreeable rhythm, the helpful impacts stretch out past the actual domain, advancing a feeling of quiet and profound prosperity. This all encompassing methodology perceives the interconnectedness of physical and psychological well-being, tending to respiratory health in a far reaching way.

Progressing flawlessly, the story presents the nourishing part of the drive — a cautiously organized dietary routine intended to supplement the helpful impacts of music. Nutritionists team up with medical services experts to distinguish key supplements fundamental for respiratory wellbeing. The subsequent dietary arrangement, plentiful in nutrients and minerals known for their lung-supporting properties, turns into a basic aspect of the all encompassing structure. This wholesome co-operative energy points not exclusively to sustain the body's interior protections yet additionally to improve the general adequacy of the Supplement rich Song Troupe.

The inclusivity of the Supplement rich Tune Group arises as a foundation of the introduction. The program is custom fitted to oblige people of fluctuating ages, foundations, and ailments. Whether a member looks for preventive measures or addresses existing respiratory difficulties, the versatile idea of the outfit guarantees a customized approach. This comprehensiveness reaches out to a pledge to openness, supporting the drive's central goal to democratize pneumonic health and make it available to different networks.

Besides, the introduction investigates the local area driven ethos of Lung Life savers' drive. The Supplement rich Tune Group rises above the bounds of a simple wellbeing program, changing into a social power that saturates networks, schools, and medical care organizations. Local area outreach drives become a point of convergence, as studios, workshops, and intelligent meetings multiply. These drives are not simple dispersal of data; they are an impetus for social change, encouraging an aggregate comprehension of respiratory wellbeing as a vital piece of by and large prosperity.

Instruction turns into a vital mainstay of Lung Helps' effort endeavors. The introduction highlights the significance of engaging people with information about respiratory wellbeing, demystifying normal confusions, and imparting a proactive way to deal with prosperity. Through coordinated efforts with schools and instructive organizations, the drive turns into a wellspring of motivation for the future, planting the seeds for a future where respiratory wellbeing is a necessary piece of the social texture.

The introduction to pneumonic health unfurls as an ensemble of development, with every component adding to an agreeable entirety. From the multifaceted subtleties of logical examination to the restorative force of music and the sustaining substance of nourishment, Lung Helps' drive remains as a demonstration of the endless capability of all encompassing ways to deal with prosperity. The preface welcomes people not exclusively to set out on an individual excursion towards respiratory wellbeing yet in addition to partake in an aggregate undertaking that rises above individual limits. It is a tribute to the interconnectedness of science, craftsmanship, and local area — an introduction that resounds with the commitment of a better and agreeable future for people and social orders the same.

1.1 Introduction to the importance of lung health

The Prologue to the significance of lung wellbeing fills in as an entryway to understanding the basic job that the respiratory framework plays in supporting generally speaking prosperity. It establishes the groundwork for an exhaustive investigation of the elements that add to ideal lung capability and, likewise, a solid and satisfying life.

In the huge scene of human life structures, the lungs arise as unrecognized yet truly great individuals, playing out an unending undertaking that is key to our reality — relaxing. The Presentation starts by enlightening the noteworthy complexities of the respiratory framework. It dives into the physical miracles of aviation routes, alveoli, and bronchioles, underscoring the intricate coordination expected for the trading of oxygen and carbon dioxide. This basic comprehension makes way for a significant enthusiasm for the significance of keeping up with respiratory wellbeing.

The story grows to highlight the complex idea of lung wellbeing, rising above its job as a simple oxygen trade system. Past its physiological capabilities, the lungs act as watchmen of generally speaking prosperity. They go about as a significant line of protection against ecological toxins, allergens, and microorganisms, assuming an essential part in resistant observation. The Presentation underlines the lungs' job in supporting life through oxygenation as well as in advancing strength against outside dangers, featuring the interconnectedness of respiratory wellbeing with the body's more extensive safeguard components.

As the significance of lung wellbeing turns out to be progressively obvious, the Acquaintance turns with the difficulties that advanced ways of life posture to respiratory prosperity. Natural contaminations, stationary propensities, and way of life factors add to a developing predominance of respiratory issues. The story dives into the effect of air contamination, smoking, and other outer stressors on lung capability, illustrating the dangers that prowl in the contemporary world. This part fills in as a source of inspiration, encouraging people to perceive the meaning of proactive measures in safeguarding and upgrading lung wellbeing.

Changing flawlessly, the story investigates the results of compromised respiratory wellbeing. Respiratory circumstances, going from normal sicknesses like asthma to constant infections like ongoing obstructive aspiratory illness (COPD), become the dominant focal point. The Presentation reveals insight into the commonness of these circumstances, their effect on day to day existence, and the related medical services trouble. This investigation fills in as a convincing inspiration for people to focus on their respiratory prosperity, perceiving the significance of preventive measures and early mediations.

Against this scenery, the story presents the idea of comprehensive respiratory health. It advocates for a shift from a responsive way to deal with respiratory wellbeing to a proactive and thorough model that incorporates way of life changes, mindfulness, and inventive intercessions. The Presentation lays the basis for the groundbreaking excursion that follows — an excursion that rises above the ordinary limits of medical care and embraces a multi-layered way to deal with prosperity.

A key topical component woven into the texture of the Presentation is the acknowledgment that lung wellbeing is certainly not a singular undertaking however a basic piece of the more extensive range of individual and local area prosperity. The interconnectedness of physical and emotional wellness, the expanding influences of natural variables on respiratory flexibility, and the shared parts of prosperity structure fundamental strings in this story. The Presentation fills in as an impetus for a change in outlook, welcoming people to see respiratory wellbeing not in segregation but rather as a vital part of an all encompassing and amicable life.

In addition, the account expects the rise of imaginative drives, for example, Lung Helps' Supplement rich Song Gathering, as guides of progress in the scene of respiratory wellbeing.

These drives mean a takeoff from customary methodologies, coordinating logical exploration, melodic treatment, and dietary science into a groundbreaking embroidery. The Presentation arouses interest about the capability of such comprehensive projects, laying the foundation for the investigation of how these intercessions can reclassify the scene of respiratory wellbeing.

Developing the establishment laid by the Prologue to the significance of lung wellbeing, the story dives further into the complexities of respiratory prosperity. It further investigates the repercussions of ecological elements, way of life decisions, and the predominance of respiratory circumstances, winding around an embroidery that features the direness of proactive measures in saving and improving lung wellbeing.

The story initially centers around the ubiquitous danger of air contamination, a contemporary test that has desperate ramifications for respiratory wellbeing. The thick transaction of toxins in the air turns into an unavoidable peril, penetrating the fragile components of the respiratory framework. The Presentation inspects the hindering impacts of breathing in particulate matter, ozone, and different contaminations, highlighting the requirement for uplifted mindfulness and coordinated endeavors to address this quiet aggressor. As urbanization and industrialization raise, the story portrays the approaching results of uncontrolled natural corruption on lung wellbeing.

At the same time, the story investigates the inescapable effect of way of life decisions on respiratory prosperity. The predominance of smoking, inactive propensities, and unfortunate dietary practices adds to a scene where respiratory issues multiply. The Presentation looks at the complex dance between way of life elements and lung wellbeing, unwinding the instruments through which smoking harms lung tissue, inactive ways of behaving compromise cardiovascular wellness, and unfortunate nourishment denies the group of indispensable supplements significant for respiratory flexibility. This investigation fills in as an obvious sign of the modifiable idea of these gamble factors, encouraging people to pursue informed decisions that can decidedly impact their lung wellbeing.

As the story disentangles the strings of ecological and way of life challenges, it consistently changes to a conversation on the predominance and effect of respiratory circumstances. From the more normal hardships like asthma to the weakening persistent circumstances like ongoing obstructive pneumonic sickness (COPD), the Presentation features the broadness of respiratory difficulties that people face. The story goes past simple measurements, digging into the lived encounters of those wrestling with respiratory circumstances, accentuating the significant effect on day to day existence, profound prosperity, and cultural investment.

In light of this mind boggling scene of difficulties, the story presents the idea of all encompassing respiratory health as an extraordinary worldview. It advocates for a proactive methodology that stretches out past the customary clinical model to include way of life changes, schooling, and imaginative intercessions.

The Presentation fills in as an impetus for a change in context, welcoming people to see their respiratory wellbeing not only as a receptive reaction to disease but rather as a proactive interest in their general prosperity.

In the midst of this investigation, the account presents Lung Helps' Supplement rich Song Outfit as a symbolic illustration of development in the field of respiratory wellbeing. This drive typifies a takeoff from customary methodologies, incorporating logical exploration, melodic treatment, and healthful science into an all encompassing structure. The Presentation arouses interest in the capability of such mediations to reclassify the scene of respiratory wellbeing. The Supplement rich Tune Group turns into an encouraging sign, outlining the conceivable outcomes that emerge when science, workmanship, and nourishment merge to make a groundbreaking ensemble of prosperity.

Moreover, the story extends its topical investigation of the interconnectedness of respiratory wellbeing with more extensive parts of life and society. The mental elements of lung wellbeing, including the effect of pressure and close to home prosperity on respiratory flexibility, come into center. The Presentation highlights the complex dance among mental and actual wellbeing, underlining the requirement for a comprehensive methodology that tends to the psyche body association. This acknowledgment turns into a basic component in the story, building up the possibility that ideal respiratory wellbeing is an agreeable exchange of different variables.

Expanding on this establishment, the story stretches out its look to the shared parts of respiratory prosperity. It perceives that lung wellbeing is certainly not a lone undertaking however an essential piece of local area wellbeing. The expanding influences of natural variables, way of life decisions, and in general prosperity stretch out past individual limits, influencing the wellbeing and imperativeness of networks. The Presentation fills in as a clarion call for aggregate activity, encouraging networks to meet up in cultivating a climate that advances respiratory health.

The story unfurls as a continuum of the Prologue to the significance of lung wellbeing. It explores through the intricacies of natural difficulties, way of life factors, and the predominance of respiratory circumstances, featuring the critical requirement for proactive measures. The account consistently advances to the groundbreaking worldview of all encompassing respiratory wellbeing, making way for the investigation of inventive intercessions like the Supplement rich Tune Troupe. As the story extends its investigation of the interconnectedness of respiratory wellbeing with more extensive parts of life and society, it turns into a source of inspiration for people and networks the same to set out on an excursion towards a better and agreeable future.

1.2 Overview of the role of nutrition in respiratory well-being

The Outline of the job of nourishment in respiratory prosperity sets out on an extensive investigation of the multifaceted association between dietary decisions and the strength of the respiratory framework. This excursion into the domain of sustenance perceives that what we consume has expansive ramifications past broad wellbeing — it fundamentally impacts the versatility and usefulness of the lungs.

To get a handle on the significant effect of nourishment on respiratory prosperity, it is basic to initially grasp the central job of the respiratory framework. The lungs, with their many-sided organization of aviation routes and alveoli, act as the door for oxygen to enter the body and carbon dioxide to be ousted. This physiological cycle is fundamental for supporting life. The Outline digs into the dietary necessities that help this intricate component, underlining the requirement for a different scope of supplements to sustain the respiratory framework.

A urgent focal point of the story is on cell reinforcements, which assume an essential part in moderating oxidative pressure — a cycle embroiled in the turn of events and movement of respiratory illnesses. The Outline features the presence of cell reinforcements in different products of the soil, exhibiting their capability to kill destructive free extremists and safeguard lung tissues. This investigation fills in as an establishment for understanding the preventive parts of nourishment in respiratory wellbeing, laying the foundation for dietary decisions that can moderate the gamble of respiratory circumstances.

At the same time, the story unfurls the meaning of nutrients and minerals in respiratory prosperity. Vital participants like L-ascorbic acid, vitamin E, and selenium arise as fundamental parts that add to the support of lung wellbeing. The Outline clarifies their jobs in collagen amalgamation, resistant capability, and cancer prevention agent safeguard, highlighting their effect on respiratory versatility. The investigation of these micronutrients turns into a demonstration of the complex exchange among sustenance and the physiological cycles that support the lungs.

The Outline broadens its look past individual supplements to the more extensive range of dietary examples. It recognizes the impact of dietary decisions, for example, the Mediterranean eating routine, which is eminent for its mitigating properties and has been related with further developed lung capability. This investigation of dietary examples turns into an entryway to figuring out the all encompassing nature of nourishment in respiratory prosperity — a cooperative energy of different supplements working in show to brace the body against respiratory difficulties.

Additionally, the account grows to address the job of explicit nutritional categories, like fish and nuts, in advancing respiratory wellbeing. Omega-3 unsaturated fats, found plentifully in fish, show mitigating properties that might help people with respiratory circumstances. Nuts, wealthy in cancer prevention agents and solid fats, add to the in general dietary profile that upholds lung capability. The Outline disentangles the healthful fortunes implanted in these nutritional categories, delineating how dietary variety can be outfit as a device for respiratory prosperity.

Changing flawlessly, the story explores through the effect of stoutness on respiratory wellbeing — a frequently neglected perspective in conversations of sustenance and lung capability. The Outline reveals insight into the unpredictable connection between overabundance weight, irritation, and the improvement of respiratory circumstances like asthma and obstructive rest apnea. This investigation highlights the requirement for all encompassing ways to deal with nourishment that address the presence of gainful supplements as well as the more extensive setting of weight the executives for ideal respiratory prosperity.

The story doesn't avoid recognizing the difficulties presented by dietary decisions that might be adverse to respiratory wellbeing. The predominance of handled food varieties, high in added substances and trans fats, and the effect of sweet refreshments come into center. The Outline looks at how these dietary examples add to irritation and oxidative pressure, laying the preparation for figuring out the job of nourishment in sustaining the respiratory framework as well as in deflecting possible damage.

As the story unfurls, the Outline presents the idea of customized nourishment — a methodology that perceives individual varieties in dietary requirements in view of hereditary, ecological, and way of life factors. This change in perspective difficulties the one-size-fits-all way to deal with sustenance, supporting for custom fitted dietary mediations that think about a singular's remarkable prerequisites for respiratory prosperity. This customized approach turns into a foundation of the story, mirroring the nuanced idea of nourishment in streamlining lung wellbeing.

The Outline recognizes that the effect of nourishment on respiratory prosperity stretches out across the life expectancy. From the urgent phases of fetal improvement to the maturing system, dietary decisions assume a significant part in forming respiratory versatility. The account investigates the ramifications of maternal sustenance on fetal lung improvement, featuring the enduring impacts that nourishing decisions during pregnancy can have on the respiratory wellbeing of the posterity. Likewise, as people age, the Outline tends to the changing wholesome necessities and the significance of adjusting dietary propensities to help respiratory capability in the later phases of life.

With regards to respiratory circumstances, the Outline offers bits of knowledge into the job of nourishment as a corresponding way to deal with customary clinical mediations.

It investigates how dietary methodologies, like mitigating diets and explicit supplement supplementation, can be incorporated into the administration of respiratory circumstances like asthma and persistent obstructive pneumonic sickness (COPD). This investigation turns into an extension between preventive sustenance and restorative nourishment, outlining the continuum of dietary mediations that can be outfit to help respiratory prosperity.

The account doesn't bind itself to the singular circle however stretches out its scope to cultural and worldwide ramifications of dietary examples. The Outline dives into the abberations in admittance to nutritious food, perceiving that financial elements impact the capacity of people and networks to pursue sound dietary decisions. This investigation turns into a source of inspiration, encouraging for aggregate endeavors to resolve foundational issues that add to dietary imbalances and, thus, differences in respiratory wellbeing.

Moreover, the story presents the idea of healthful instruction as an impetus for engaging people to go with informed dietary decisions. The Outline highlights the significance of cultivating wholesome education, outfitting people with the information and abilities to explore the intricate scene of food decisions. This instructive aspect turns into a necessary piece of the story, accentuating that the effect of sustenance on respiratory prosperity isn't exclusively dependent upon the accessibility of nutritious food yet in addition on the capacity of people to go with informed decisions.

Expanding upon the fundamental investigation of sustenance in respiratory prosperity, this story further tests the transaction of dietary variables with irritation — a focal subject in the complicated connection among nourishment and lung wellbeing. Irritation, frequently saw as a two sided deal, is a characteristic reaction to injury or disease. In any case, when constant and uncontrolled, it can turn into a contributing element to different respiratory circumstances. The Outline digs into the components by which nourishment can regulate irritation, offering bits of knowledge into dietary methodologies that hold guarantee in cultivating respiratory strength.

The account unfurls by clarifying the idea of provocative pathways and their suggestions for respiratory wellbeing. Provocative cycles are complicatedly connected to the movement of respiratory circumstances like asthma, ongoing bronchitis, and COPD. The Outline explores through the sub-atomic scene, investigating how explicit supplements can either fuel or relieve aggravation. The job of omega-3 unsaturated fats, tracked down in overflow in greasy fish, flaxseeds, and pecans, arises as a central participant in this regulation, exhibiting their capability to hose provocative reactions inside the respiratory framework.

In addition, the Outline looks at the effect of dietary fats on irritation, causing to notice the harmony between omega-3 and omega-6 unsaturated fats. While omega-3 unsaturated fats display calming properties, an excess of omega-6 unsaturated fats, frequently pervasive in handled and seared food varieties, can add to a provocative milieu.

This investigation extends the comprehension of how dietary decisions impact the fragile balance between favorable to provocative and calming powers inside the body.

Cell reinforcements, a common topic in conversations of nourishment and respiratory wellbeing, reemerge with regards to irritation. The Outline disentangles the cell reinforcement's part in killing free revolutionaries — a cycle basic to forestalling oxidative pressure and constant irritation. The overflow of cell reinforcements in organic products, vegetables, and entire grains turns into a key part in the story, stressing the requirement for dietary variety to tackle the full range of these defensive mixtures.

The story flawlessly advances to an investigation of the stomach lung hub, a many-sided association between the gastrointestinal and respiratory frameworks. The Outline enlightens how the stomach microbiota, affected by dietary decisions, can influence aggravation in the lungs. Dietary fiber, prebiotics, and probiotics arise as crucial components in sustaining a reasonable and various stomach microbiome. This investigation highlights the all encompassing nature of sustenance, where decisions reach out past individual supplements to shape the advantageous connection among stomach and lung wellbeing.

With regards to aggravation and respiratory circumstances, the Outline presents the capability of mitigating eats less. These dietary examples, wealthy in natural products, vegetables, entire grains, and lean proteins, have been related with diminished aggravation and worked on respiratory results. The Outline turns into a manual for understanding how dietary decisions can be decisively adjusted to make a calming milieu inside the body, cultivating a climate that upholds lung wellbeing.

As the story unfurls, the Outline digs into the idea of wholesome immunomodulation — a unique exchange among nourishment and the resistant framework. The safe framework, complicatedly associated with provocative cycles, assumes a focal part in protecting the respiratory framework against microbes and keeping up with homeostasis. The Outline investigates the effect of key supplements, like vitamin D, zinc, and selenium, in tweaking resistant reactions and upgrading the body's capacity to safeguard against respiratory dangers.

The investigation of immunomodulation reaches out to the impact of explicit dietary examples, like the Mediterranean eating routine, on resistant capability. Wealthy in cell reinforcements, mitigating fats, and a different cluster of supplements, the Mediterranean eating regimen turns into a worldview for saddling the synergistic impacts of sustenance on resistant and respiratory wellbeing. The Outline highlights the extraordinary capability of dietary examples that go past separated supplements, encouraging an all encompassing way to deal with enhancing lung capability.

The story further develops its investigation by tending to the job of hydration in respiratory prosperity. Sufficient liquid admission is pivotal for keeping up with the bodily fluid layer coating the aviation routes, which fills in as a defensive obstruction against respiratory aggravations. The Outline underlines the meaning of remaining very much hydrated as a major part of respiratory consideration, featuring water as a fundamental supplement that adds to the general soundness of the respiratory framework.

As the account develops, the Outline recognizes the significance of overcoming any issues between dietary science and clinical practice. It investigates the joining of wholesome mediations into the administration of respiratory circumstances, stressing the potential for customized nourishment plans custom-made to the special necessities of people. This convergence of sustenance and clinical consideration turns into a boondocks where proof based dietary methodologies can supplement conventional clinical methodologies, making ready for a more far reaching and integrative model of respiratory wellbeing.

Past individual contemplations, the account stretches out its look to the more extensive cultural ramifications of sustenance in respiratory prosperity. The Outline perceives the job of general wellbeing drives in forming dietary examples at the populace level. It turns into a source of inspiration for policymakers and medical services experts to focus on dietary training and intercessions that address foundational issues adding to respiratory wellbeing inconsistencies.

The Outline of the job of nourishment in respiratory prosperity crosses a diverse scene, unwinding the complicated associations between dietary decisions and lung wellbeing. From the balance of irritation to immunomodulation, the story investigates how sustenance can be bridled as a device to streamline respiratory flexibility. The Outline turns into a manual for exploring the intricacies of dietary examples, underscoring the comprehensive idea of sustenance in cultivating lung wellbeing. It requires a change in perspective where nourishing mediations reach out past individual supplements to envelop customized plans, mitigating eats less carbs, and a cultural obligation to healthful schooling. In this extensive excursion, the Outline turns into an impetus for changing the story around respiratory prosperity, welcoming people, medical services experts, and policymakers to perceive the groundbreaking capability of nourishment in molding a better and agreeable future.

1.3 Brief exploration of common lung ailments and their connection to diet

A concise investigation of normal lung sicknesses and their association with diet uncovers a nuanced transaction between respiratory wellbeing and nourishing decisions. Respiratory circumstances like asthma, constant obstructive pneumonic illness (COPD), and bronchitis frequently have complex etiologies, including a mix of hereditary inclination, natural elements, and way of life decisions, including diet.

Asthma, a constant fiery state of the aviation routes, is described by episodes of wheezing, windedness, and chest snugness. While hereditary qualities and natural triggers assume a critical part in asthma improvement, arising research proposes that dietary elements may likewise impact asthma chance and seriousness. The Outline dives into the effect of cancer prevention agents, tracked down in products of the soil, on moderating oxidative pressure — a basic consider asthma. Also, the story investigates the expected job of omega-3 unsaturated fats, present in greasy fish and certain plant sources, in balancing irritation and upgrading lung capability, offering bits of knowledge into dietary techniques that might supplement customary asthma the board.

Persistent obstructive pneumonic infection (COPD), an ever-evolving lung condition that incorporates constant bronchitis and emphysema, is frequently connected to long haul openness to aggravations, for example, tobacco smoke and air contamination. Notwithstanding, the job of diet in COPD is acquiring consideration as specialists investigate the likely effect of explicit supplements on illness movement. The Outline explores through the impact of cell reinforcements and calming fats in moderating COPD-related aggravation, revealing insight into dietary examples that might offer remedial advantages. Also, the account investigates the results of ailing health in COPD patients, accentuating the significance of wholesome help in improving respiratory capability and by and large prosperity.

Bronchitis, an irritation of the bronchial cylinders, can be intense or ongoing. It frequently emerges from viral or bacterial diseases, openness to aggravations, and smoking. While irresistible specialists are essential supporters of bronchitis, the Outline analyzes how dietary decisions can impact the body's insusceptible reaction. Cell reinforcements and resistant helping supplements become central focuses, displaying the capability of a supplement rich eating regimen in supporting the body's capacity to battle diseases and decrease the seriousness and term of bronchitis episodes.

The story stretches out its investigation to cystic fibrosis, a hereditary problem that principally influences the respiratory and stomach related frameworks. People with cystic fibrosis experience thick and tacky bodily fluid in their aviation routes, prompting repetitive lung contaminations and respiratory difficulties. The Outline enlightens the wholesome contemplations in cystic fibrosis the board, stressing the requirement for a fatty eating regimen to fulfill the expanded energy needs connected with the condition. Pancreatic protein supplements, fat-solvent nutrients, and thoughtfulness regarding generally wholesome status become necessary parts of the dietary way to deal with cystic fibrosis.

As the story digs into the association between normal lung sicknesses and diet, it recognizes the double job of nourishment — both as a preventive measure and as a correlative restorative system.

The Outline highlights that while dietary decisions may not act as independent therapies for respiratory circumstances, they can assume a critical part in improving by and large lung wellbeing, decreasing the gamble of intensifications, and supporting regular clinical mediations.

Moreover, the Outline investigates the effect of weight on respiratory wellbeing and the likely job of diet in corpulence related lung conditions. Heftiness, described by abundance body weight, has been related with an expanded gamble of creating respiratory issues like asthma, rest apnea, and weakened lung capability. The story explores through the components connecting stoutness and respiratory wellbeing, featuring the job of irritation, hormonal elements, and mechanical weight on the respiratory framework. Dietary examples that advance weight the executives and address fundamental metabolic variables become key contemplations in the comprehensive way to deal with respiratory prosperity.

The story doesn't avoid recognizing the difficulties presented by specific dietary examples that might fuel respiratory circumstances. For example, the utilization of exceptionally handled food sources, wealthy in added substances and trans fats, is related with expanded irritation and oxidative pressure. Sweet drinks, connected to stoutness and metabolic aggravations, likewise come into center. The Outline turns into a manual for perceiving and addressing dietary decisions that might add to respiratory difficulties, stressing the significance of a decent and wellbeing advancing eating routine.

With regards to cellular breakdown in the lungs, the Outline recognizes the multifactorial idea of the illness, with smoking being the essential gamble factor. Notwithstanding, arising research recommends that particular dietary elements might impact cellular breakdown in the lungs hazard and forecast. Cell reinforcements, phytochemicals, and certain nutrients and minerals tracked down in natural products, vegetables, and entire grains are investigated for their likely defensive impacts. The story turns into a course for understanding how dietary examples wealthy in these defensive mixtures might add to an all encompassing system for cellular breakdown in the lungs counteraction and the board.

The story further investigates the capability of plant-based eats less carbs in respiratory wellbeing. Plant-based consumes less calories, portrayed by an accentuation on natural products, vegetables, entire grains, and vegetables while limiting or taking out creature items, have been related with mitigating and cell reinforcement impacts. The Outline turns into a focal point through which the advantages of plant-based slims down are inspected, offering bits of knowledge into how such dietary examples might add to respiratory prosperity.

Additionally, the account addresses the job of hydration in supporting respiratory wellbeing. Sufficient liquid admission is fundamental for keeping up with the bodily fluid layer in the aviation routes, which fills in as a defensive boundary against respiratory aggravations.

The Outline highlights the significance of remaining very much hydrated as a key part of respiratory consideration, featuring water as a fundamental supplement that adds to the general soundness of the respiratory framework.

Developing the investigation of normal lung illnesses and their association with diet, the story brings a more profound jump into explicit supplements and dietary examples that hold guarantee in advancing respiratory wellbeing. The Outline turns into an exhaustive aide, winding through the perplexing embroidery of nourishment and respiratory prosperity, tending to both preventive and restorative perspectives.

One vital part of the account is the investigation of the job of cancer prevention agents in lung wellbeing. Cancer prevention agents, including nutrients C and E, beta-carotene, and selenium, assume a significant part in killing free revolutionaries and relieving oxidative pressure — a cycle involved in the turn of events and worsening of respiratory circumstances. The Outline digs into the dietary wellsprings of these cell reinforcements, underlining the significance of a brilliant and shifted diet wealthy in natural products, vegetables, nuts, and seeds. By unwinding the defensive impacts of cell reinforcements, the story highlights how dietary decisions can act as a strong safeguard against oxidative harm to the respiratory framework.

Additionally, the story investigates the capability of omega-3 unsaturated fats in respiratory prosperity. Tracked down in greasy fish, flaxseeds, chia seeds, and pecans, omega-3 unsaturated fats are perceived for their calming properties. The Outline turns into a passage to understanding how these fundamental fats can tweak irritation in the aviation routes, possibly lessening the seriousness of side effects in respiratory circumstances like asthma and COPD. The incorporation of omega-3-rich food varieties into the eating regimen arises as an essential dietary way to deal with tackling the mitigating potential for respiratory strength.

The account stretches out its investigation to the perplexing connection between diet, aggravation, and the stomach microbiome. Dietary fiber, prebiotics, and probiotics become heroes in this story, impacting the creation and variety of the stomach microbiota. The Outline explores through the bidirectional correspondence between the stomach and lungs, stressing how a solid stomach microbiome can add to safe guideline and irritation tweak in the respiratory framework. Matured food sources, high-fiber decisions, and the development of a different microbiome arise as dietary procedures with potential expansive consequences for respiratory wellbeing.

With regards to respiratory circumstances like asthma, the Outline investigates the possible advantages of explicit dietary examples. The Mediterranean eating regimen, portrayed by a wealth of organic products, vegetables, entire grains, nuts, and olive oil, turns into a point of convergence.

This dietary example, known for its mitigating and cancer prevention agent properties, lines up with rules that may emphatically impact asthma results. The story digs into the parts of the Mediterranean eating regimen, offering bits of knowledge into how this all encompassing way to deal with nourishment can be bridled to help respiratory prosperity.

Besides, the Outline tends to the significance of keeping a solid load with regards to respiratory wellbeing. Stoutness, frequently connected with an expanded gamble of respiratory circumstances and weakened lung capability, comes into center. The account explores through the instruments connecting weight and respiratory difficulties, featuring the job of aggravation, hormonal elements, and mechanical weight on the respiratory framework. Dietary examples that focus on weight the executives and metabolic wellbeing become necessary parts of the comprehensive way to deal with respiratory prosperity.

The story stretches out its investigation to the likely advantages of plant-based eats less carbs in respiratory wellbeing. Plant-based consumes less calories, described by an emphasis on natural products, vegetables, entire grains, and vegetables while limiting or wiping out creature items, are related with calming and cell reinforcement impacts. The Outline turns into a focal point through which the story inspects how such dietary examples might add to respiratory prosperity. By unwinding the expected defensive impacts of plant-based eats less carbs, the story offers a comprehensive viewpoint on the job of nourishment in advancing lung wellbeing.

Notwithstanding the investigation of dietary examples, the Outline dives into the significance of customized nourishment in streamlining respiratory prosperity. Perceiving the fluctuation in individual reactions to dietary mediations, the story turns into a promoter for custom fitted methodologies that consider hereditary, natural, and way of life factors. The arising field of nutrigenomics, which investigates the cooperation among nourishment and hereditary qualities, turns into a point of convergence. The account highlights the potential for customized nourishment intends to address individual weaknesses and tackle the full range of dietary intercessions for respiratory wellbeing.

As the account unfurls, it tends to the significance of hydration in supporting respiratory wellbeing. Sufficient liquid admission is essential for keeping up with the bodily fluid layer in the aviation routes, which fills in as a defensive boundary against respiratory aggravations. The Outline highlights the meaning of remaining very much hydrated as a major part of respiratory consideration, featuring water as a fundamental supplement that adds to the general wellbeing of the respiratory framework.

Additionally, the account investigates the possible job of nourishing mediations in the administration of ongoing respiratory circumstances. While recognizing the focal job of clinical medicines, the story turns into a scaffold between regular consideration and corresponding wholesome procedures.

From calming diets to designated supplement supplementation, the Outline offers bits of knowledge into how dietary intercessions might be coordinated into the extensive administration of conditions like asthma and COPD. This investigation turns into a demonstration of the developing scene of respiratory consideration, perceiving the possible cooperative energies between ordinary medication and sustenance.

The extended investigation of normal lung illnesses and their association with diet portrays the perplexing connections among sustenance and respiratory prosperity. From cancer prevention agents and omega-3 unsaturated fats to the Mediterranean eating routine and customized sustenance, the account explores through the assorted scene of dietary methodologies. The Outline fills in as an aide, offering experiences into how dietary decisions can serve both preventive and helpful jobs in advancing lung wellbeing. It highlights the capability of sustenance as a dynamic and fundamental part of respiratory consideration, perceiving the groundbreaking effect that educated dietary decisions can have on the direction of respiratory prosperity. As the story grows the material of understanding, it welcomes people, medical care experts, and scientists to investigate the tremendous capability of nourishment in molding a better and amicable future for respiratory wellbeing.

Chapter 2

The Antioxidant Overture
Blueberries

The Cell reinforcement Suggestion: Blueberries

In the tremendous ensemble of nourishment, the blueberry becomes the dominant focal point as a virtuoso, winding around a cell reinforcement suggestion that reverberates with potential medical advantages. These little, lively berries, having a place with the Vaccinium class, have procured their status as a nourishing force to be reckoned with, enamoring both taste buds and logical interest. As the Cell reinforcement Suggestion unfurls, it dives into the rich woven artwork of blueberries, investigating their dietary structure, cancer prevention agent properties, and the multi-layered manners by which they add to generally speaking prosperity.

Blueberries are adored for their magnificent eruption of flavor as well as for their amazing supplement profile. The Cancer prevention agent Suggestion starts by unwinding the dietary extravagance of these small diamonds. Blueberries are low in calories yet high in fundamental supplements, making them a supplement thick expansion to a decent eating routine. They are a rich wellspring of nutrients, especially L-ascorbic acid and vitamin K, and give a significant portion of dietary fiber, which is instrumental in supporting stomach related wellbeing.

The account explores through the variety of micronutrients present in blueberries, stressing their job in bracing the body with fundamental components.

At the core of the Cell reinforcement Suggestion lies the investigation of blueberries as a cancer prevention agent force to be reckoned with. Cell reinforcements are intensifies that kill free revolutionaries, shaky atoms that can cause cell harm and add to different constant illnesses. Blueberries brag a range of cell reinforcements, with anthocyanins becoming the dominant focal point. Anthocyanins, answerable for the particular blue shade of the berries, are strong flavonoids that have been broadly read up for their cell reinforcement and mitigating properties. The account unwinds the defensive impacts of anthocyanins, accentuating their true capacity in moderating oxidative pressure and irritation inside the body.

As the Cell reinforcement Suggestion unfurls, it dives into the components by which blueberries apply their cancer prevention agent impacts. The account investigates how these berries go past simple cancer prevention agent rummaging to regulate cell flagging pathways and quality articulation. Blueberries arise as powerful entertainers in the cell ensemble, affecting cycles that manage irritation, safe capability, and oxidative equilibrium. The story turns into an excursion into the unpredictable dance between blueberry cancer prevention agents and the cell ensemble, representing the profundity of their effect on cell wellbeing.

In addition, the Cell reinforcement Suggestion stretches out its investigation to the possible advantages of blueberries in advancing cardiovascular wellbeing. The cardiovascular framework, defenseless against oxidative pressure and irritation, stands to acquire from the cancer prevention agent ability of blueberries. The story explores through research featuring the job of blueberries in lessening circulatory strain, further developing lipid profiles, and upgrading endothelial capability. Blueberries become a delightful expansion to the eating routine as well as a strong partner in keeping up with cardiovascular prosperity.

The Cell reinforcement Suggestion winds around a story string interfacing blueberries to mental wellbeing. As the maturing populace develops, worries about mental deterioration become progressively huge. Blueberries, with their rich anthocyanin content, become heroes in the journey for cerebrum wellbeing. The story investigates studies proposing that standard blueberry utilization might be connected to enhancements in mental capability, memory, and security against age-related mental degradation. The many-sided interchange between blueberry cell reinforcements and brain connections turns into a point of convergence, featuring their true capacity as mind helping berries.

With regards to the Cell reinforcement Suggestion, the story stretches out its investigation to the likely job of blueberries in diabetes the executives. Diabetes, portrayed by debilitated insulin capability and raised glucose levels, is a worldwide wellbeing concern.

The cancer prevention agent properties of blueberries, especially their effect on insulin responsiveness, come into center. The story explores through research proposing that blueberry utilization might add to more readily glucose control and diminished insulin obstruction. Blueberries become a wonderful treat as well as a dietary partner in the perplexing dance of glucose guideline.

The Cell reinforcement Suggestion turns into a culinary investigation as it digs into the flexibility of blueberries in the kitchen. From breakfast parfaits to servings of mixed greens, smoothies, and sweets, blueberries flawlessly coordinate into different dishes. The account commends the availability of blueberries, making it practical for people to integrate these cell reinforcement rich berries into their everyday culinary collection. The energetic varieties and kinds of blueberries become an encouragement to investigate innovative and nutritious culinary undertakings, highlighting that ideal wellbeing can be both scrumptious and outwardly engaging.

The account stretches out its look to the capability of blueberries in skin wellbeing, a viewpoint frequently ignored in conversations of nourishment. The cell reinforcement properties of blueberries, especially their part in battling oxidative pressure, add to the skin's flexibility against ecological harm. The Cell reinforcement Suggestion turns into an excursion into the complicated connection among blueberries and skin wellbeing, featuring their true capacity in advancing a brilliant and energetic composition. Blueberries, with their anthocyanin-rich sythesis, become a treat for the taste buds as well as a supporting remedy for the skin.

Also, the Cell reinforcement Suggestion recognizes the expected job of blueberries in aggravation balance. Ongoing irritation, a sign of different infections, is a complex organic reaction that can be impacted by dietary decisions. Blueberries, with their calming properties, become instrumental players in the orchestra of irritation guideline. The story investigates how blueberries might add to lessening irritation at the sub-atomic level, giving experiences into their true capacity as dietary mediations in the administration of fiery circumstances.

The Cell reinforcement Suggestion turns into a festival of blueberries as a practical and open superfood. The development of blueberries, with their versatility to different environments, adds to their far and wide accessibility. The story recognizes the possible job of blueberry development in advancing reasonable food frameworks, underscoring the ecological advantages of a harvest that flourishes in different horticultural settings. Blueberries become a nourishing force to be reckoned with as well as an image of the interconnectedness between dietary decisions, ecological manageability, and worldwide prosperity.

As the Cell reinforcement Suggestion arrives at its crescendo, it turns into a source of inspiration — a greeting for people to embrace blueberries as a delightful and wellbeing elevating expansion to their eating regimens. The story highlights that the excursion to ideal wellbeing is certainly not a performance try however a cooperative exertion among people and the lively range of supplements tracked down in entire food varieties.

Blueberries, with their cell reinforcement ensemble, entice people to investigate the plentiful universe of supplement rich, plant-based food varieties that can add to an agreeable and fortifying life.

climax of the perplexing story woven around these minuscule yet strong berries. The investigation stretches out to the capability of blueberries in malignant growth avoidance and treatment. Malignant growth, a mind boggling and diverse gathering of sicknesses, has earned broad examination consideration in regards to the expected job of diet in its turn of events and movement. The Cell reinforcement Suggestion turns into a manual for grasping how blueberries, with their rich exhibit of cell reinforcements and bioactive mixtures, may add to the complicated dance of malignant growth counteraction and backing.

Blueberries, as the account unfurls, arise as likely partners in the battle against disease. The cell reinforcements present in blueberries, especially anthocyanins, quercetin, and resveratrol, become central focuses in the investigation of their enemy of disease properties. The account explores through examinations proposing that these mixtures might impact different systems related with disease improvement, including oxidative pressure, irritation, and the guideline of cell development and apoptosis. Blueberries become a superb expansion to the plate as well as a food with the possibility to add to an extensive technique for malignant growth counteraction.

With regards to explicit kinds of disease, the Cell reinforcement Suggestion investigates the likely advantages of blueberries in battling colorectal malignant growth. Colorectal disease, with its multifaceted transaction of hereditary and ecological variables, turns into a point of convergence in the story. The investigation stretches out to studies recommending that the cell reinforcements and fiber in blueberries might add to a diminished gamble of colorectal disease and deal expected defensive impacts. Blueberries, with their complex way to deal with wellbeing, become a delightful nibble as well as a dietary part with suggestions for colorectal malignant growth counteraction.

Moreover, the Cell reinforcement Suggestion digs into the possible job of blueberries in supporting the resistant framework — a basic player in disease observation and guard. The story investigates how the cancer prevention agents in blueberries might add to safe tweak, upgrading the body's capacity to perceive and kill strange cells. The unpredictable connection between nourishment, safe capability, and malignant growth turns into a focal subject, representing how blueberries might have an impact in bracing the body's regular guards against carcinogenic cells.

As the story unfurls, it tends to the subtleties of integrating blueberries into different dietary examples. Whether consumed new, frozen, or as a feature of culinary manifestations, blueberries offer flexibility that lines up with various dietary inclinations.

The Cell reinforcement Suggestion turns into a culinary aide, motivating people to investigate the horde manners by which blueberries can be incorporated into feasts and tidbits. The account praises the availability of blueberries, underscoring that the excursion to ideal wellbeing can be both pleasant and comprehensive.

Additionally, the Cell reinforcement Suggestion recognizes the possible job of blueberries in metabolic wellbeing — a perspective unpredictably connected to conditions like stoutness and type 2 diabetes. The account investigates studies proposing that the cell reinforcements and bioactive mixtures in blueberries might impact metabolic pathways, adding to further developed insulin responsiveness and glucose guideline. Blueberries become a magnificent expansion to the eating routine as well as a possible partner in the far reaching way to deal with metabolic prosperity.

In the more extensive setting of the story, the Cell reinforcement Suggestion turns into a festival of the collaboration among blueberries and other supplement rich food sources. The story investigates how blueberries can be essential for a comprehensive dietary example that incorporates a different cluster of natural products, vegetables, entire grains, and lean proteins. The investigation turns into a demonstration of the likely advantages of a decent and shifted diet, featuring the cooperative impacts of supplements working in show to advance by and large wellbeing and prosperity.

Besides, the Cancer prevention agent Suggestion explores through the capability of blueberries in advancing stomach wellbeing — a viewpoint progressively perceived for its suggestions on in general prosperity. The story investigates how the cell reinforcements and fiber in blueberries might add to a decent and different stomach microbiome. The complicated transaction between nourishment, the stomach microbiota, and different parts of wellbeing turns into a focal topic, showing how blueberries might assume a part in cultivating stomach strength and supporting stomach related wellbeing.

The story grows its investigation to the possible advantages of blueberries in alleviating age-related mental degradation. Maturing, with its related mental difficulties, turns into a point of convergence in the story. The Cell reinforcement Suggestion turns into an excursion into research proposing that the cell reinforcements and bioactive mixtures in blueberries might add to mental versatility and further developed mind capability in more established grown-ups. Blueberries, with their possible neuroprotective impacts, become a great expansion to the eating routine as well as a food with suggestions for mental prosperity.

As the story arrives at its pinnacle, it turns into a reflection on the more extensive ramifications of blueberries for general wellbeing. The Cell reinforcement Suggestion turns into a source of inspiration, encouraging people, medical services experts, and policymakers to perceive the capability of blueberries in advancing wellbeing and forestalling illness.

The story highlights the significance of incorporating supplement rich food varieties like blueberries into general wellbeing drives, underlining the extraordinary effect that educated dietary decisions can have on a populace's prosperity.

The Cell reinforcement Suggestion of blueberries winds around a far reaching story, investigating the multi-layered manners by which these berries add to wellbeing and prosperity. From their cell reinforcement ability to likely advantages in disease avoidance, metabolic wellbeing, safe help, and mental versatility, blueberries arise as lively supporters of the orchestra of sustenance. The story turns into a greeting for people to embrace the extravagance of blueberries as a feature of a fair and shifted diet, perceiving their capability to upgrade by and large wellbeing. As the story closes, it becomes a festival of blueberries as well as a recognition for the many-sided transaction among sustenance and the coordination of an amicable and stimulating life.

2.1 In-depth examination of the powerful antioxidants in blueberries

The top to bottom Assessment of the Strong Cell reinforcements in Blueberries

Blueberries, those little and tasty berries, are not just an eruption of pleasantness on the sense of taste; they are a healthful mother lode, overflowing with powerful cell reinforcements. As we set out on a top to bottom assessment of the strong cell reinforcements in blueberries, we disentangle the perplexing natural chemistry and wellbeing advancing properties that make these berries a striking expansion to a fair and healthy eating regimen.

At the core of the investigation lies an appreciation for the assorted exhibit of cancer prevention agents tracked down in blueberries. These cell reinforcements, intensifies that kill free revolutionaries and alleviate oxidative pressure, incorporate flavonoids, polyphenols, and, most quite, anthocyanins. Anthocyanins, liable for the energetic blue and purple tints of blueberries, arise as the stars of the cell reinforcement gathering. The inside and out assessment explores through the atomic design of anthocyanins, revealing insight into their astounding skill to search free extremists and give defensive advantages to cell wellbeing.

The cell reinforcement excursion of blueberries brings us into the domain of flavonoids, a class of mixtures celebrated for their cell reinforcement and mitigating properties. The top to bottom assessment investigates the unpredictable subcategories of flavonoids present in blueberries, for example, quercetin, myricetin, and kaempferol. Every one of these flavonoids, with its one of a kind substance structure, adds to the cell reinforcement orchestra that unfurls inside the berries. The story turns into an excursion into the sub-atomic subtleties of flavonoids, representing their part in balancing cell cycles and supporting generally speaking wellbeing.

Besides, the top to bottom assessment stretches out its look to polyphenols — a wide class of phytochemicals bountiful in blueberries. Polyphenols, with their different designs and works, add to the cell reinforcement and calming impacts of blueberries. The account explores through the polyphenolic scene, investigating how these mixtures collaborate with cell pathways, impact quality articulation, and add to the multi-layered benefits credited to blueberries. The top to bottom assessment turns into an exhaustive investigation of polyphenols as basic players in the cell reinforcement symphony of blueberries.

The investigation develops as we dig into the potential medical advantages of the cell reinforcements in blueberries. The top to bottom assessment tends to oxidative pressure — a lopsidedness between free extremists and cancer prevention agents that can add to cell harm and different persistent illnesses. Blueberries, with their rich cancer prevention agent content, become heroes in the account of moderating oxidative pressure. The account investigates studies recommending that the cell reinforcements in blueberries might add to decreasing oxidative harm to cells and tissues, offering possible defensive impacts against conditions like cardiovascular sickness, neurodegenerative issues, and disease.

With regards to cardiovascular wellbeing, the top to bottom assessment turns into an excursion into the systems by which blueberry cell reinforcements might present advantages to the heart and veins. The account investigates studies showing that the cancer prevention agents in blueberries might add to further developing circulatory strain, decreasing irritation, and upgrading endothelial capability. Blueberries, with their capability to emphatically impact cardiovascular gamble factors, become a tasty expansion to the eating routine as well as a dietary methodology for supporting heart wellbeing.

Moreover, the top to bottom assessment stretches out its investigation to the possible neuroprotective impacts of blueberry cell reinforcements. Neurodegenerative issues, described by the ever-evolving loss of nerve cells, stand out with regards to blueberry research. The account dives into studies recommending that the cell reinforcements in blueberries, especially anthocyanins, may apply defensive impacts on the cerebrum. The investigation turns into an excursion into the unpredictable transaction among blueberries and mental wellbeing, delineating their true capacity in supporting mind capability and possibly relieving age-related mental deterioration.

In the domain of disease counteraction and treatment, the top to bottom assessment turns into a complete investigation of how blueberry cell reinforcements might impact cell processes pertinent to carcinogenesis. The story explores through examinations recommending that the cell reinforcements in blueberries might add to decreasing the gamble of specific malignant growths by adjusting irritation, affecting cell cycle guideline, and advancing apoptosis — the modified demise of harmed cells. Blueberries arise as likely partners in the complicated scene of malignant growth counteraction, exhibiting their complex way to deal with supporting by and large wellbeing.

Notwithstanding their job in ongoing sickness counteraction, the top to bottom assessment turns into a culinary investigation, praising the capability of blueberries as flexible and tasty increments to different dishes. Whether consumed new, frozen, or integrated into recipes going from servings of mixed greens and smoothies to sweets and sauces, blueberries offer culinary flexibility that lines up with assorted dietary inclinations. The account highlights the openness of blueberries, making it plausible for people to embrace these cancer prevention agent rich berries as a component of their day to day culinary collection.

Also, the top to bottom assessment recognizes the expected advantages of blueberries in supporting metabolic wellbeing — a perspective significant with regards to conditions like stoutness and type 2 diabetes. The account investigates studies recommending that the cell reinforcements in blueberries might impact metabolic pathways, adding to further developed insulin responsiveness and glucose guideline. Blueberries, with their capability to decidedly affect metabolic markers, become a brilliant expansion to the eating regimen as well as a dietary partner in the exhaustive way to deal with metabolic prosperity.

The investigation stretches out to the likely advantages of blueberries in advancing stomach wellbeing — a region progressively perceived for its suggestions on generally prosperity. The top to bottom assessment digs into studies proposing that the cell reinforcements and fiber in blueberries might add to a fair and various stomach microbiome. The story turns into an excursion into the multifaceted transaction between sustenance, the stomach microbiota, and different parts of wellbeing, representing how blueberries might assume a part in cultivating stomach strength and supporting stomach related wellbeing.

Moreover, the top to bottom assessment investigates the expected job of blueberries in safe balance — a viewpoint urgent for by and large wellbeing and illness avoidance. The account explores through examinations recommending that the cell reinforcements in blueberries might add to upgrading safe capability, furnishing the body with added versatility against contaminations and sicknesses. Blueberries become a tasty treat as well as a dietary part with suggestions for supporting the body's regular safeguard systems.

As the inside and out assessment arrives at its climax, it turns into a reflection on the more extensive ramifications of blueberries for general wellbeing. The story highlights the capability of blueberries to add to a supplement rich and cell reinforcement pressed diet, perceiving the groundbreaking effect that educated dietary decisions can have on a populace's prosperity. Blueberries, with their openness and culinary flexibility, become images of the interconnectedness between individual dietary decisions, general wellbeing drives, and the advancement of a better and stronger society.

The investigation of the strong cancer prevention agents in blueberries develops as we dive into the complicated exchange between these bioactive mixtures and cell processes. The top to bottom assessment turns into an excursion into the sub-atomic ensemble organized by blueberry cell reinforcements, representing their dynamic effect on wellbeing and prosperity.

Anthocyanins, the colors answerable for the energetic tones of blueberries, become heroes in the story of cancer prevention agent power. These water-solvent mixtures, having a place with the flavonoid family, go past their job as simple colorants. The top to bottom assessment digs into studies proposing that anthocyanins have astounding cell reinforcement and calming properties, adding to their true capacity in advancing cardiovascular wellbeing, diminishing oxidative pressure, and relieving aggravation. The story turns into a festival of anthocyanins as central participants in the cell reinforcement gathering of blueberries.

The investigation stretches out to quercetin, a flavonoid plentifully tracked down in blueberries. Quercetin, commended for its cell reinforcement and mitigating impacts, turns into a point of convergence in the top to bottom assessment. The story explores through the capability of quercetin in regulating cell flagging pathways, affecting quality articulation, and adding to the multi-layered benefits credited to blueberries. Quercetin arises as a flexible cell reinforcement with suggestions for cardiovascular wellbeing, safe balance, and the possible counteraction of constant sicknesses.

Additionally, the top to bottom assessment investigates the possible collaboration between various cell reinforcements in blueberries. The story turns into an excursion into the cooperative impacts of anthocyanins, quercetin, and other polyphenols present in blueberries. Studies propose that the blend of cancer prevention agents might make added substance or synergistic impacts, improving their general effect on cell wellbeing. The investigation turns into a demonstration of the intricacy and concordance inside the cell reinforcement ensemble of blueberries, delineating how the different cluster of bioactive mixtures works in show to advance ideal wellbeing.

In the domain of cell assurance, the story tends to the job of blueberry cancer prevention agents in fighting oxidative pressure. Oxidative pressure, coming about because of an awkwardness between free extremists and cancer prevention agents, is embroiled in the improvement of different constant sicknesses. The top to bottom assessment turns into a manual for understanding how the cancer prevention agents in blueberries go about as scroungers of free revolutionaries, killing these responsive particles and forestalling cell harm. Blueberries arise as protectors of cell honesty, offering a powerful safeguard against the harmful impacts of oxidative pressure.

Moreover, the account stretches out its investigation to the likely calming impacts of blueberry cell reinforcements.

Constant irritation, a tireless and second rate insusceptible reaction, is connected to the improvement of various illnesses, including cardiovascular circumstances, neuro-degenerative problems, and certain tumors. The top to bottom assessment turns into an excursion into studies recommending that the cell reinforcements in blueberries might tweak fiery pathways, diminishing the development of favorable to provocative particles and advancing a calming climate inside the body. Blueberries become flavorful augmentations to the eating regimen as well as dietary partners in the continuous fight against persistent irritation.

With regards to cardiovascular wellbeing, the inside and out assessment turns into a nearer investigation of how blueberry cell reinforcements might impact key cardiovascular gamble factors. The story digs into studies demonstrating that the cell reinforcements in blueberries might add to further developing lipid profiles by decreasing degrees of LDL cholesterol and fatty substances. Moreover, blueberries might upgrade endothelial capability, supporting the wellbeing and adaptability of veins. The investigation turns into an excursion into the capability of blueberries to emphatically influence factors related with cardiovascular sicknesses, situating them as dietary supporters of heart wellbeing.

Besides, the top to bottom assessment tends to the likely advantages of blueberry cell reinforcements in advancing mental wellbeing. Neurodegenerative issues, described by the dynamic loss of nerve cells, definitely stand out enough to be noticed with regards to blueberry research. The story explores through examinations recommending that the cancer prevention agents in blueberries might cross the blood-cerebrum boundary, applying defensive consequences for synapses and impacting mental capability. Blue-berries become superb treats for the taste buds as well as likely partners in the journey for mental flexibility and the avoidance old enough related mental deterioration.

In the unpredictable scene of malignant growth avoidance and treatment, the story turns into an investigation of how blueberry cancer prevention agents might impact cell processes pertinent to carcinogenesis. The top to bottom assessment explores through examinations showing that the cell reinforcements in blueberries might add to lessening the gamble of specific tumors by balancing flagging pathways related with cell development, apoptosis, and aggravation. Blueberries arise as expected players in the mind boggling and dynamic field of disease avoidance, exhibiting their diverse way to deal with supporting generally wellbeing.

Notwithstanding their possible job in constant sickness counteraction, the story turns into a culinary festival, featuring the flexibility and openness of blueberries. The inside and out assessment recognizes that integrating blueberries into the eating regimen isn't just a wellbeing cognizant decision yet additionally a delightful and charming one. Whether consumed new, frozen, or as fixings in different recipes, blueberries become a culinary pleasure that lines up with assorted preferences and inclinations. The story turns into a greeting for people to investigate the culinary capability of blueberries, relishing both their taste and wellbeing advancing properties.

Moreover, the top to bottom assessment recognizes the possible advantages of blueberries in supporting metabolic wellbeing — a perspective significant with regards to conditions like heftiness and type 2 diabetes. The story investigates studies proposing that the cancer prevention agents in blueberries might impact metabolic pathways, adding to further developed insulin responsiveness and glucose guideline. Blueberries become a wonderful expansion to the eating routine as well as a possible partner in the thorough way to deal with metabolic prosperity.

The investigation reaches out to the likely advantages of blueberries in advancing stomach wellbeing — a region progressively perceived for its suggestions on by and large prosperity. The top to bottom assessment digs into studies recommending that the cell reinforcements and fiber in blueberries might add to a fair and different stomach microbiome. The story turns into an excursion into the multifaceted transaction between sustenance, the stomach microbiota, and different parts of wellbeing, showing how blueberries might assume a part in cultivating stomach strength and supporting stomach related wellbeing.

Additionally, the account investigates the likely job of blueberries in resistant tweak — a perspective significant for in general wellbeing and sickness avoidance. The top to bottom assessment explores through examinations recommending that the cell reinforcements in blueberries might add to improving safe capability, furnishing the body with added versatility against contaminations and diseases. Blueberries become a delightful treat as well as a dietary part with suggestions for supporting the body's normal guard instruments.

As the top to bottom assessment arrives at its peak, it turns into a reflection on the more extensive ramifications of blueberries for general wellbeing. The story highlights the capability of blueberries to add to a supplement rich and cell reinforcement pressed diet, perceiving the extraordinary effect that educated dietary decisions can have on a populace's prosperity. Blueberries, with their openness and culinary flexibility, become images of the interconnectedness between individual dietary decisions, general wellbeing drives, and the advancement of a better and stronger society.

The top to bottom assessment of the strong cell reinforcements in blueberries disentangles a story that goes past the pleasantness of these berries. From anthocyanins and flavonoids to polyphenols, blueberries arise as an orchestra of cell reinforcements that add to different parts of wellbeing. The story turns into a greeting for people to see the value in the complex natural chemistry of blueberries, perceiving their expected in supporting cardiovascular wellbeing, mental capability, malignant growth counteraction, metabolic prosperity, stomach wellbeing, and resistant regulation. As the story closes, it becomes a festival of blueberries as well as a recognition for the significant effect that these cell reinforcement rich berries can have on the orchestra of human wellbeing.

2.2 Recipes and tips for incorporating blueberries into a lung-friendly diet

Recipes and Ways to integrate Blueberries into a Lung-Accommodating Eating routine

The excursion toward respiratory prosperity frequently includes comprehensive way of life decisions, and nourishment assumes a crucial part in supporting lung wellbeing. Blueberries, with their cell reinforcement rich profile and different medical advantages, arise as a tasty partner in making a lung-accommodating eating regimen. This investigation digs into recipes and tips that flawlessly incorporate blueberries into a respiratory-cognizant culinary collection, making it a dietary change as well as a flavorful and energizing culinary experience.

Blueberry and Spinach Smoothie:

Fixings:

1 cup new or frozen blueberries

1 cup new spinach leaves

1/2 banana

1/2 cup Greek yogurt

1/2 cup almond milk

1 tablespoon chia seeds

Ice 3D squares (discretionary)

Directions:

In a blender, consolidate blueberries, spinach, banana, Greek yogurt, almond milk, and chia seeds.

Mix until smooth and rich.

Whenever wanted, add ice 3D squares and mix again for a reviving chill.

Fill a glass and partake in a supplement stuffed smoothie that joins the cell reinforcement force of blueberries with the lung-accommodating advantages of spinach.

Blueberry Quinoa Salad:

Fixings:
1 cup cooked quinoa, cooled
1 cup new blueberries
1/2 cup cucumber, diced
1/4 cup red onion, finely cleaved
1/4 cup feta cheddar, disintegrated
2 tablespoons new mint, cleaved
2 tablespoons extra-virgin olive oil
1 tablespoon balsamic vinegar
Salt and pepper to taste

Guidelines:
In an enormous bowl, join cooked quinoa, blueberries, cucumber, red onion, feta cheddar, and new mint.

In a little bowl, whisk together olive oil, balsamic vinegar, salt, and pepper.

Sprinkle the dressing over the quinoa combination and throw tenderly to consolidate.

Serve chilled as a reviving and supplement thick side dish or quick bite.

Blueberry and Pecan Cereal:

Fixings:
1/2 cup moved oats
1 cup almond milk
1/2 cup new blueberries
2 tablespoons cleaved pecans
1 tablespoon honey
1/2 teaspoon cinnamon

Directions:
In a pot, join moved oats and almond milk.

Cook over medium intensity, blending at times, until the oats are delicate and the combination has thickened.

Mix in new blueberries and keep on cooking for an extra 2-3 minutes until the blueberries are warmed.

Eliminate from intensity and move the oats to a bowl.

Top with slashed pecans, shower with honey, and sprinkle with cinnamon.

Partake in a generous and lung-accommodating breakfast that consolidates the fiber-rich decency of oats with the cell reinforcement influence of blueberries and the omega-3 unsaturated fats in pecans.

Blueberry and Salmon Plate of mixed greens:

Fixings:
1 cup blended salad greens
4 ounces barbecued or prepared salmon, chipped
1/2 cup new blueberries

1/4 cup cherry tomatoes, split

1/4 cup cut cucumber

1/4 cup red chime pepper, daintily cut

1 tablespoon olive oil

1 tablespoon balsamic vinegar

Salt and pepper to taste

Directions:

Orchestrate blended salad greens on a plate.

Top with chipped salmon, new blueberries, cherry tomatoes, cut cucumber, and red ringer pepper.

In a little bowl, whisk together olive oil, balsamic vinegar, salt, and pepper.

Shower the dressing over the plate of mixed greens not long prior to serving.

Partake in a lung-accommodating and protein-rich plate of mixed greens that consolidates the calming advantages of salmon with the cell reinforcement extravagance of blueberries.

Ways to integrate Blueberries into a Lung-Accommodating Eating routine:

Nibble on New Blueberries: Keep a bowl of new blueberries effectively open for a fast and helpful tidbit. Their normal pleasantness fulfills desires while giving a portion of cell reinforcements.

Add Blueberries to Yogurt: Blend new or frozen blueberries into your number one yogurt for a delectable and supplement pressed nibble. Greek yogurt, specifically, adds an additional protein support.

Blueberry Salsa: Make an energetic salsa utilizing new blueberries, diced tomatoes, red onion, cilantro, lime juice, and a dash of jalapeño. Serve it as a fixing for barbecued chicken or fish.

Blueberry Chia Pudding: Consolidate blueberries with chia seeds and almond milk to make a nutritious and fiber-rich pudding. Allow it to sit for the time being in the cooler for a helpful breakfast or nibble choice.

Blueberry Tea: Inject your number one home grown tea with blueberries for a delightful and cell reinforcement rich refreshment. Add a sprinkle of lemon for an invigorating turn.

Blueberry and Pecan Prepared Products: Integrate blueberries and cleaved pecans into natively constructed biscuits, flapjacks, or waffles for a lung-accommodating breakfast choice.

Blueberry and Kale Salad: Join new blueberries with kale, almonds, and a light vinaigrette dressing for a supplement thick and cell reinforcement stuffed salad.

Blueberry Smoothie Bowls: Make dynamic smoothie bowls by mixing blueberries with different organic products, yogurt, and a dash of honey. Top with granola, nuts, and seeds for added surface.

Blueberry Oat Bars: Heat oat bars with a blueberry filling for a healthy and versatile bite. These bars can be ready ahead of time for a helpful in a hurry choice.

Blueberry and Dull Chocolate Path Blend: Make a lung-accommodating path blend by joining blueberries in with dim chocolate lumps, almonds, and pumpkin seeds. Segment it into little compartments for a fantastic tidbit.

Integrating blueberries into a lung-accommodating eating routine includes imagination and an eagerness to investigate different culinary choices. From breakfast to tidbits and principal feasts, blueberries can be consistently incorporated into various dishes, offering both flavor and medical advantages. Likewise with any dietary change, it's fundamental to think about individual inclinations and talk with medical care experts or nutritionists for customized guidance on making a lung-accommodating eating routine that lines up with explicit wellbeing needs. At last, embracing the flexibility of blueberries can change dietary decisions into a magnificent and empowering venture toward respiratory prosperity.

Blueberry and Avocado Smoothie Bowl:

Fixings:

1 cup frozen blueberries

1/2 ready avocado

1/2 cup spinach leaves

1/2 cup coconut water

1 tablespoon chia seeds

Fixings: cut banana, granola, and a shower of honey

Directions:

In a blender, consolidate frozen blueberries, ready avocado, spinach leaves, coconut water, and chia seeds.

Mix until smooth and rich.

Empty the smoothie into a bowl.

Top with cut banana, granola, and a shower of honey.

Partake in a supplement stuffed and outwardly engaging smoothie bowl that consolidates the cell reinforcement force of blueberries with the rich surface of avocado.

Blueberry and Almond Short-term Oats:

Fixings:

1/2 cup moved oats

1/2 cup almond milk

1/4 cup new blueberries

1 tablespoon almond spread

1 teaspoon maple syrup

Fixings: cut almonds and extra blueberries

Guidelines:

In a container or holder, join moved oats, almond milk, new blueberries, almond spread, and maple syrup.

Mix well, it are completely covered to guarantee the oats.

Cover and refrigerate for the time being.

In the first part of the day, give the oats a decent mix.

Top with cut almonds and extra blueberries.

Partake in a helpful and lung-accommodating breakfast that joins the dietary decency of oats, almonds, and blueberries.

Blueberry and Ginger Mixed Water:

Fixings:

1 cup new blueberries

1-inch piece of ginger, cut

1 liter water

Ice 3D shapes

Discretionary: mint leaves for embellish

Directions:

In a pitcher, consolidate new blueberries and cut ginger.

Fill the pitcher with water.

Refrigerate for a couple of hours to permit the flavors to implant.

Add ice 3D shapes prior to serving.

Discretionary: Trimming with mint leaves for a reviving turn.

Taste on this hydrating and cell reinforcement rich implanted water over the course of the day.

Blueberry and Pecan Stuffed Chicken Bosom:

Fixings:

2 boneless, skinless chicken bosoms

1/2 cup new blueberries

1/4 cup cleaved pecans

1 tablespoon balsamic vinegar

1 tablespoon olive oil

Salt and pepper to taste

New rosemary for embellish

Guidelines:

Preheat the broiler to 375°F (190°C).

In a bowl, join new blueberries, cleaved pecans, balsamic vinegar, olive oil, salt, and pepper.

Make a pocket in every chicken bosom and stuff them with the blueberry and pecan combination.

Season the beyond the chicken bosoms with extra salt and pepper.

Place the stuffed chicken bosoms in a baking dish.

Heat for 25-30 minutes or until the chicken is cooked through.

Decorate with new rosemary prior to serving.

Partake in a flavorful and protein-rich fundamental dish that consolidates the exquisite notes of chicken with the pleasantness of blueberries.

Ways to integrate Blueberries into a Lung-Accommodating Eating regimen (Proceeded):

Blueberry and Greek Yogurt Parfait: Make a basic yet fulfilling parfait by layering new blueberries with Greek yogurt and a sprinkle of granola. This brilliant treat can act as a nutritious breakfast or a healthy pastry.

Blueberry and Green Tea Smoothie: Mix blueberries with prepared green tea, a sprinkle of almond milk, and a dash of honey for a reviving and cell reinforcement rich smoothie. This blend saddles the medical advantages of the two blueberries and green tea.

Blueberry and Turkey Wrap: Develop a lung-accommodating wrap by filling an entire grain tortilla with cut turkey, new blueberries, spinach leaves, and a bit of hummus. Roll it up for a heavenly and compact lunch choice.

Blueberry and Basil Vinaigrette: Raise your servings of mixed greens with a custom made vinaigrette. Mix new blueberries with balsamic vinegar, olive oil, and new basil for a tasty dressing that upgrades the healthful profile of your greens.

Blueberry and Curds Bowl: Join new blueberries with curds for a fast and protein-pressed nibble. Add a sprinkle of nuts or seeds for added crunch and healthy benefit.

Blueberry and Lemon Biscuits: Prepare natively constructed biscuits utilizing entire grain flour, new blueberries, and a sprinkle of lemon zing for a great treat. These biscuits can be delighted in as a tidbit or a faultless pastry.

Blueberry and Pecan Omelet: Upgrade your morning omelet by consolidating new blueberries and slashed pecans. This exquisite and sweet blend adds an eruption of flavor to your morning meal.

Blueberry and Chocolate Smoothie: Enjoy your sweet desires with a nutritious chocolate and blueberry smoothie. Mix frozen blueberries with cocoa powder, banana, and almond milk for a righteous pastry roused treat.

Blueberry and Feta Quinoa Bowl: Make a flavorful quinoa bowl by consolidating cooked quinoa with new blueberries, disintegrated feta cheddar, and a sprinkle of olive oil. This exceptional mix offers a brilliant mix of flavors and surfaces.

Blueberry and Fish Salad: Redesign your fish salad by adding new blueberries, celery, and a light Greek yogurt dressing. This curve on an exemplary gives an explosion of newness and cell reinforcement goodness.

Integrating blueberries into a lung-accommodating eating routine stretches out past the kitchen — it's an excursion of culinary inventiveness and cognizant decisions that focus on respiratory prosperity. These recipes and tips exhibit the flexibility of blueberries, showing the way that they can be flawlessly incorporated into different dishes over the course of the day. Whether delighted in smoothies, mixed greens, primary courses, or tidbits, blueberries contribute their tasty flavor as well as their cell reinforcement rich profile, making them an important expansion to a lung-cognizant culinary collection.

2.3 Personal stories of individuals benefiting from blueberry-rich nutrition

Individual Accounts of People Profiting from Blueberry-Rich Nourishment

In the domain of nourishing decisions, the effect of integrating blueberries into one's eating routine goes past logical examinations and wellbeing proposals — it resounds in the individual accounts of people who significantly affect their prosperity. These accounts offer looks into the existences of individuals who have embraced blueberry-rich nourishment and saw positive changes in different parts of their wellbeing.

Sarah's Excursion to Heart Wellbeing:

Sarah, a 45-year-old mother of two, had forever been aware of keeping a sound way of life, yet her new cholesterol levels were a reason to worry. Regardless of a reasonable eating regimen and standard activity, her LDL cholesterol stayed raised. Looking for a characteristic methodology, Sarah chose to remember more blueberries for her everyday feasts in the wake of finding out about their likely cardiovascular advantages.

Throughout a while, Sarah integrated blueberries into her morning smoothies, mixed greens, and tidbits. The outcomes were shocking — her subsequent cholesterol test uncovered a huge diminishing in LDL cholesterol levels. Sarah credits this positive change to the cell reinforcements in blueberries, which are known for their part in supporting heart wellbeing.

"Blueberries turned into my unmistakable advantage against elevated cholesterol. Besides the fact that they added an eruption of flavor to my feasts, yet they likewise assumed a urgent part in working on my cardiovascular markers. It's extraordinary how something so straightforward and scrumptious can have such a significant effect in your wellbeing," Sarah shares.

Jason's Mental Lift:

For Jason, a 60-year-old retired person, mental degradation was a worry that incited him to investigate dietary intercessions. In the wake of finding out about the possible mental advantages of blueberries, he chose to make them an everyday staple in his eating regimen. Jason integrated new blueberries into his morning meal, delighted in them as a tidbit, and, surprisingly, tried different things with adding them to exquisite dishes.

Over the long run, Jason saw enhancements in his mental capability and memory. He felt more keen, more engaged, and encountered a feeling of mental clearness that he hadn't felt in years. While he recognizes that different way of life factors add to mental wellbeing, Jason solidly accepts that the standard consideration of blueberries assumed a critical part in his mental prosperity.

"I had some doubts from the get go, yet the progressions I encountered were certain. Blueberries turned into my mind fuel, and I could feel the distinction in my day to day existence. It's ameliorating to know that something so tasty is additionally feeding my brain," Jason reflects.

Elena's Excursion to Destroy Versatility:

Elena, a 30-year-old promoting proficient, battled with stomach related issues that frequently left her inclination swelled and awkward. Looking for a characteristic arrangement, she went to the expected advantages of blueberries for stomach well-being. Captivated by studies proposing that the cell reinforcements and fiber in blueberries could uphold a fair stomach microbiome, Elena chose to explore different avenues regarding integrating blueberries into her feasts.

She began her day with a blueberry and yogurt parfait, remembered blueberries for her plates of mixed greens, and, surprisingly, mixed them into her morning smoothies. Bit by bit, Elena saw a positive change in her stomach related prosperity. The bulging decreased, and she felt more agreeable after dinners. Elena credits these enhancements to the stomach accommodating properties of blueberries, which turned into a foundation of her stomach related wellbeing venture.

"Blueberries turned into my partners in the fight against stomach related uneasiness. The more I found out about their likely effect on the stomach, the more I needed to investigate ways of remembering them for my feasts. It's astounding the way in which something so little can have such a major effect by they way you feel," Elena shares.

Imprint's Athletic Presentation Upgrade:

Mark, a 35-year-old wellness fan, was generally keeping watch for ways of improving his athletic execution. While he followed a restrained preparation routine, he looked for a dietary edge that could supplement his wellness objectives. Captivated by the cell reinforcement and calming properties of blueberries, Imprint chose to coordinate them into his pre-and post-exercise dinners.

He remembered blueberries for his protein smoothies, matched them with Greek yogurt for a recuperation tidbit, and, surprisingly, tried different things with integrating them into energy bars. Mark saw enhancements in his recuperation time, decreased muscle touchiness, and a general lift in his energy levels. Blueberries turned into a staple in his wellness nourishment, contributing not exclusively to his actual prosperity yet additionally to the happiness regarding his feasts.

"Blueberries turned into my go-to when it came to supporting my exercises. I could feel the distinction in how rapidly my body recuperated, and the additional explosion of flavor made my feasts more charming. It's a basic yet strong expansion to my wellness process," Imprint communicates.

Sophie's Invulnerable Strength:

Sophie, a 28-year-old medical care proficient, wound up continually engaging occasional sicknesses because of her rushed plan for getting work done. Looking for ways of improving her resistant flexibility, Sophie went to the invulnerable adjusting properties of blueberries. She began integrating blueberries into her everyday daily practice, frequently getting a charge out of them as a bite or adding them to her morning oats.

To her pleasure, Sophie saw a diminishing in the recurrence of her sicknesses. Her resistant framework appeared to be more powerful, and she felt far improved prepared to deal with the requests of her work. Sophie credits blueberries for assuming a crucial part in supporting her safe wellbeing and thinks of them as a non-debatable piece of her health schedule.

"Blueberries turned into my reinforcement against successive diseases. Working in medical care, I really wanted something to support my safe framework, and blueberries ended up being the ideal expansion. Realizing that I'm supporting my wellbeing with something so delectable is a mutual benefit," Sophie reflects.

Tom's Weight The board Achievement:

Tom, a 40-year-old dad of three, battled with keeping a sound load notwithstanding his endeavors to consistently work-out. Roused by the possible metabolic advantages of blueberries, Tom chose to integrate them into his dinners as a feature of his weight the executives system. He remembered blueberries for his morning smoothies, prepared them into plates of mixed greens, and, surprisingly, explored different avenues regarding involving them in flavorful recipes.

Over the long run, Tom saw a continuous and supportable decline in his weight. While he recognizes that general way of life changes assumed a part, he accepts that the consideration of blueberries added to his prosperity. Tom keeps on partaking in the flexibility of blueberries in his feasts, seeing them as a delightful part of his continuous weight the executives venture.

"Blueberries turned into my partners in the excursion toward a better weight. They added pleasantness to my dinners without the culpability, and I could see the positive effect on my general prosperity. A little change had a major effect in my life," Tom shares.

Laura's Sweet Process to Metabolic Congruity:

Laura, a 32-year-old educator and mother of two, confronted difficulties with fluctuating energy levels and incidental sugar desires. Worried about the effect of her eating regimen on her metabolic wellbeing, she went to blueberries as a sweet yet nutritious other option. Laura began integrating blueberries into her morning oats, mixing them into smoothies, and in any event, getting a charge out of them as a faultless treat.

As she embraced this blueberry-rich methodology, Laura saw balanced out energy levels and diminished desires for sweet tidbits. She credits these positive changes to the regular pleasantness of blueberries, combined with their fiber content, which added to a more adjusted and amicable metabolic experience.

"Blueberries turned into my sweet getaway from the high points and low points of energy crashes. I love that I can fulfill my sweet tooth without undermining my prosperity. It resembles having somewhat explosion of happiness in each chomp," Laura shares.

David's Joint Wellbeing Renewal:

David, a 50-year-old IT proficient, had been wrestling with joint inconvenience that frequently influenced his everyday exercises. Captivated by the calming properties of blueberries, he chose to investigate their true capacity in advancing joint wellbeing.

David integrated blueberries into his day to day daily practice, getting a charge out of them in yogurt bowls, sprinkling them on oats, and in any event, integrating them into exquisite dishes.

After some time, David saw a decrease in joint distress and expanded adaptability. While he kept on following other joint-accommodating practices, like standard activity and keeping a solid weight, he accepts that the expansion of blueberries assumed a significant part in renewing his joint wellbeing.

"Blueberries turned into my partners in the excursion toward joint solace. I could feel the distinction in my everyday exercises, and it's consoling to know that something so flavorful is additionally supporting my joints from the inside," David reflects.

Sophia's Skin Brilliance Reestablishment:

Sophia, a 25-year-old promoting proficient, looked for a characteristic way to deal with improve the brilliance of her skin. Mindful of the job cell reinforcements play in skin wellbeing, she went to blueberries as a skincare mysterious. Sophia integrated blueberries into her eating regimen, making cancer prevention agent rich smoothie bowls, adding them to servings of mixed greens, and in any event, exploring different avenues regarding blueberry-implanted water.

As weeks passed, Sophia saw a noticeable improvement in her skin's brilliance and surface. She ascribes this shine to the cancer prevention agent force of blueberries, which added to her skin's restoration from the back to front. For Sophia, blueberries turned into a wonderful expansion to her excellence schedule, demonstrating that sustaining the skin can be both flavorful and viable.

"Blueberries turned into my excellence help. I love the way they make my skin gleam, and the way that they're so flexible in recipes is a reward. It resembles giving my skin a treat from within," Sophia communicates.

Mike's Fight Against Oxidative Pressure:

Mike, a 45-year-old business visionary, had a quick moving existence that frequently exposed him to elevated degrees of stress. Worried about the likely effect of oxidative weight on his general wellbeing, he went to blueberries as a dietary procedure. Mike remembered blueberries for his everyday daily schedule, appreciating them as tidbits, mixing them into cancer prevention agent rich smoothies, and in any event, integrating them into plates of mixed greens.

As he embraced this blueberry-rich way of life, Mike saw a feeling of strength against the impacts of pressure. While he kept on executing pressure the board rehearses, he accepts that the cell reinforcements in blueberries assumed a part in supporting his body's protection against oxidative pressure.

"Blueberries turned into my everyday portion of flexibility. In the hustle of life, realizing that I'm feeding my body with something so strong provides me with a feeling of certainty. It's a little yet significant decision for my general prosperity," Mike shares.

Emma's Excursion to Hormonal Concordance:

Emma, a 35-year-old yoga teacher, experienced hormonal changes that impacted her state of mind and generally prosperity. Captivated by the potential hormonal-adjusting impacts of blueberries, she chose to integrate them into her eating routine. Emma delighted in blueberries in her morning smoothie bowls, blended them into yogurt, and, surprisingly, remembered them for chemical well disposed recipes.

Over the long run, Emma saw a more adjusted mind-set and expanded by and large prosperity. While she proceeded with her yoga pursue and other way of life routines, she accepts that the expansion of blueberries assumed a steady part in her excursion to hormonal congruity.

"Blueberries turned into my partners in tracking down balance. I could feel the distinction by they way I moved toward every day, and it's engaging to realize that I'm pursuing decisions that line up with my prosperity, all around," Emma reflects.

An Embroidery of Changes

These individual stories weave an embroidery of changes, displaying the different ways people have embraced blueberry-rich nourishment and experienced positive changes in their wellbeing. From metabolic concordance and joint wellbeing rejuvenation to skin brilliance reestablishment, the fight against oxidative pressure, and the excursion to hormonal congruity, blueberries have become something beyond a natural product — they have become partners chasing all encompassing prosperity.

While these stories give looks into individual encounters, it's fundamental to recognize that the effect of blueberries is important for an exhaustive way of life approach. Integrating blueberries into one's eating regimen is definitely not a particular arrangement yet a delightful and nutritious part that lines up with more extensive wellbeing cognizant decisions.

As these individual stories keep on unfurling, they highlight the significant association between dietary decisions and generally prosperity. Blueberries, with their cell reinforcement rich profile and flexible culinary allure, stand as images of strengthening — an update that the excursion to better wellbeing can be both delightful and extraordinary.

As people across various different backgrounds keep on finding the advantages of blueberry-rich nourishment, these accounts become reference points of motivation. They welcome others to investigate the capability of integrating blueberries into their own lives, finding the pleasure of their flavor as well as the possible effect on different features of wellbeing. In this continuous story of prosperity, blueberries sparkle as energetic supporters of a better and really satisfying life.

Chapter 3

Omega-3 Symphony
Salmon's Respiratory Resonance

Omega-3 Ensemble: Salmon's Respiratory Reverberation

In the agreeable symphony of nourishment, where every supplement assumes an unmistakable part in supporting wellbeing, omega-3 unsaturated fats arise as a strong and fundamental piece. Among the different wellsprings of omega-3s, salmon stands apart as a virtuoso, contributing not exclusively to cardiovascular wellbeing yet in addition assuming a special part in the ensemble of respiratory prosperity. This investigation digs into the multifaceted association between omega-3 unsaturated fats found in salmon and their effect on respiratory wellbeing, uncovering the musical exchange that unfurls inside the body.

The Omega-3 Suggestion: Figuring out the Essentials

Prior to diving into the respiratory reverberation of salmon, it is basic to comprehend the fundamental components of omega-3 unsaturated fats.

Omega-3s are a class of polyunsaturated fats known for their various medical advantages, especially in supporting cardiovascular and cerebrum wellbeing. The three essential kinds of omega-3 unsaturated fats incorporate alpha-linolenic corrosive (ALA), eicosapentaenoic corrosive (EPA), and docosahexaenoic corrosive (DHA).

While ALA is found in plant-based sources, for example, flaxseeds and pecans, EPA and DHA are overwhelmingly obtained from greasy fish like salmon. These long-chain unsaturated fats assume urgent parts in different physiological capabilities, and their importance reaches out to the multifaceted dance of respiratory prosperity.

Salmon's Omega-3 Aria: EPA and DHA as one

Salmon, frequently alluded to as a healthful force to be reckoned with, becomes the dominant focal point in the omega-3 orchestra. Its wealth in both EPA and DHA positions it as a central participant in the respiratory reverberation that unfurls inside the human body. The agreement starts with EPA, known for its strong calming properties. With regards to respiratory wellbeing, irritation assumes a critical part, frequently adding to conditions like asthma and constant obstructive pneumonic infection (COPD).

Studies have recommended that the calming impacts of EPA might assist with alleviating irritation in the aviation routes, offering help to people wrestling with respiratory circumstances. The musical notes of EPA stretch out past irritation, impacting the development of particular supportive of settling middle people (SPMs) that guide in the goal of irritation — a critical viewpoint in the administration of respiratory illnesses.

DHA, the subsequent development in salmon's omega-3 aria, contributes its own arrangement of harmonies to respiratory prosperity. Plentiful in the cell layers of the lungs, DHA assumes a part in keeping up with film ease and security. This underlying scaffolding is crucial to lung capability, guaranteeing that the respiratory surfaces stay adaptable and responsive. Besides, DHA shows cell reinforcement properties, going about as a safeguard against oxidative pressure — a natural power that can influence lung wellbeing adversely.

The Respiratory Song: Salmon and Asthma The board

As the omega-3 orchestra proceeds, a striking crescendo arises with regards to asthma the executives. Asthma, a constant respiratory condition described via aviation route irritation and bronchoconstriction, presents an intricate exchange of incendiary middle people. Salmon's rich creation of EPA and DHA turns into a remedial song, impacting the organization of variables engaged with asthma pathogenesis.

Studies investigating the connection between omega-3 unsaturated fats and asthma have demonstrated that an eating regimen bountiful in these fundamental fats, especially from greasy fish like salmon, may present defensive impacts.

EPA's mitigating properties are remembered to tweak the fiery reaction in the aviation routes, possibly lessening the seriousness of asthma side effects. Moreover, the capacity of omega-3s to create SPMs adds to the goal of irritation, offering a nuanced way to deal with asthma the executives.

While the exact systems are still subjects of continuous exploration, the omega-3 ensemble, with salmon as an unmistakable soloist, introduces itself as a likely adjunctive treatment in the all encompassing administration of asthma. Integrating salmon into the eating regimen might turn into an amicable song that reverberates with those looking for regular roads to supplement standard asthma mediations.

Persistent Lung Song: Salmon's Part in COPD

Persistent obstructive pneumonic sickness (COPD), an ever-evolving respiratory condition frequently connected with ongoing bronchitis and emphysema, presents an alternate development in the omega-3 orchestra. Here, the calming and underlying scaffolding presented by EPA and DHA in salmon become featured discussions in tending to the persistent idea of the illness.

In people with COPD, the constant irritation in the aviation routes and the oxidative pressure related with the condition add to a steady decrease in lung capability.

Salmon's omega-3 aria, with its calming and cancer prevention agent rhythm, holds guarantee in moderating the fiery weight and offering underlying help to the lungs.

Research investigating the job of omega-3s, particularly from marine sources like salmon, in COPD the board proposes possible advantages. EPA's mitigating impacts might assist with lightening side effects, while DHA's underlying scaffolding turns out to be particularly important in keeping up with the honesty of lung layers. As the omega-3 ensemble unfurls, salmon's reverberation in the COPD song turns into a helpful tune that fits with traditional ways to deal with improve respiratory prosperity.

Pneumonic Preface: Salmon in Cellular breakdown in the lungs Anticipation

Past constant respiratory circumstances, the omega-3 ensemble highlighting salmon stretches out its melodic impact to the domain of cellular breakdown in the lungs avoidance. Cellular breakdown in the lungs, a mind boggling sickness with multifactorial starting points, acquaints another topical component with the creation. While omega-3 unsaturated fats are not a solution for cellular breakdown in the lungs, arising research proposes an expected job in lessening the gamble and supporting generally lung wellbeing.

The calming properties of EPA, joined with its impact on the goal of irritation through SPMs, may add to a microenvironment less helpful for the turn of events and movement of malignant cells. DHA's cell reinforcement ability adds one more layer of insurance, countering oxidative pressure and possibly decreasing the probability of cell harm that can prompt malignant growth.

Albeit the scene of omega-3s in cellular breakdown in the lungs counteraction is as yet developing, salmon's presence in this orchestra offers a nuanced and comprehensive way to deal with supporting lung wellbeing. Combined with other way of life factors, for example, keeping away from tobacco smoke and keeping a solid eating routine, the omega-3 song turns into a preventive rhythm that reverberates with those looking to sustain their respiratory guards.

Congruity in the Microbial City: Salmon, Omega-3s, and the Stomach Lung Hub

The omega-3 orchestra, with salmon as a highlighted soloist, broadens its reverberation past the lungs, venturing into the mind boggling biological system of the stomach. The stomach lung hub, a bidirectional correspondence framework between the gastrointestinal plot and the respiratory framework, adds a layer of intricacy to the melodic interchange of sustenance and wellbeing.

Salmon's omega-3 creation adds to the amicability in this microbial city. The calming impacts of EPA and DHA resound through the stomach, affecting the equilibrium of the microbiota. A dysregulated stomach microbiome has been connected to different respiratory circumstances, and the omega-3 ensemble, by advancing a sound stomach climate, in a roundabout way upholds respiratory prosperity.

Research investigating the stomach lung pivot recommends that the calming and immunomodulatory impacts of omega-3s might stretch out to the respiratory framework by regulating the stomach microbiome. Salmon's rich omega-3 piece turns into a wholesome rhythm that reverberations through this interconnected orchestra, encouraging an amicable connection between the stomach and the lungs.

Exploring the Ocean of Dietary Decisions: Useful Hints for Salmon Co-ordination

As the omega-3 ensemble including salmon unfurls its intricate yet gorgeous arrangement, reasonable contemplations become possibly the most important factor for those trying to integrate this healthful virtuoso into their eating regimens. Exploring the ocean of dietary decisions requires a harmony between culinary pleasure and wellbeing cognizant choices.

Regular Devotion to Greasy Fish: Expect to incorporate greasy fish like salmon in your eating routine no less than a few times each week. This recurrence guarantees a predictable stock of omega-3 unsaturated fats, adding to the musical notes that help respiratory wellbeing.

Changed Arrangements for Sense of taste Joy: Investigate assorted culinary arrangements to keep your sense of taste locked in. Barbecued, heated, poached, or smoked — salmon fits different cooking techniques, permitting you to relish its flavors in various ways.

Matching with Produce Flair: Upgrade the healthful effect of your salmon dishes by matching them with vivid and cancer prevention agent rich leafy foods. The ensemble of flavors and supplements intensifies the respiratory reverberation of your dinner.

Careful Decisions in Obtaining: Choose wild-got salmon whenever the situation allows. Wild-got assortments frequently have a better omega-3 profile contrasted with their homestead raised partners. Also, consider maintainable obtaining practices to line up with moral and natural contemplations.

Consolidating Omega-3 Colleagues: Extend the omega-3 ensemble by integrating different wellsprings of these fundamental unsaturated fats into your eating routine. Flaxseeds, chia seeds, pecans, and green growth based supplements are incredible side-kicks that add to the in general nourishing arrangement.

Meeting with Culinary Counselors: Look for direction from nutritionists or culinary specialists to find creative ways of remembering salmon for your dinners. From heavenly marinades to inventive side dishes, their skill can raise your culinary involvement in salmon.

Exploring the Ocean of Dietary Decisions: Viable Tips for Salmon Mix (Proceeded)

Adjusting Macronutrients for Healthy Nourishment: Consider the generally macronutrient organization of your feasts. Matching salmon with complex starches, for example, quinoa or yams, and different vegetables guarantees a fair and healthy dietary profile. This improves the satiety of your feast as well as adds to the orchestra of supplements supporting your respiratory wellbeing.

Careful Cooking Techniques for Most extreme Supplement Maintenance: Pick cooking strategies that safeguard the nourishing trustworthiness of salmon. While barbecuing and baking are famous decisions, consider delicate strategies like steaming or poaching to limit supplement misfortune. These techniques assist with holding the omega-3 unsaturated fats and other fundamental supplements that add to the respiratory reverberation of your feast.

Inventive Culinary Investigation with Worldwide Flavors: Investigate world-wide foods to imbue imagination into your salmon-based feasts. From Japanese miso-coated salmon to Mediterranean-style barbecued salmon, each culinary custom brings special flavors and fixings that supplement the omega-3 ensemble. This culinary investigation enhances your sense of taste as well as acquaints different supplements with help respiratory prosperity.

Blending Omega-3s with Generally Dietary Examples: Coordinate salmon into a balanced and different eating regimen. While omega-3s are fundamental, they are essential for a more extensive nourishing scene. Embracing dietary examples like the Mediterranean or Run (Dietary Ways to deal with Stop Hypertension) diet, which underscore various supplement rich food sources, further upgrades the musical inter-action of supplements supporting respiratory wellbeing.

Modifying Parts for Individual Necessities: Designer the piece sizes of salmon to meet individual dietary requirements and inclinations. Whether as the highlight of a dinner or a correlative fixing in servings of mixed greens and bowls, changing segments considers adaptability in integrating salmon into a reasonable eating routine. This customization guarantees that the omega-3 orchestra lines up with individual healthful objectives.

Investigating Culinary Joint efforts for Delightful Excursions: Team up with individual food devotees, cooks, or nutritionists to trade culinary thoughts and find better approaches to appreciate salmon. Partaking in cooking classes or participating in web-based networks gave to culinary investigation encourages a feeling of shared energy for nutritious and scrumptious feasts revolved around salmon's omega-3 lavishness.

Resounding Past the Plate: Way of life Contemplations for Respiratory Prosperity

While salmon's omega-3 aria becomes the overwhelming focus in the ensemble of respiratory prosperity, recognizing the all encompassing nature of health is urgent. Way of life contemplations past dietary decisions assume fundamental parts in supporting ideal respiratory capability. These contemplations fit with the dietary rhythm of salmon, adding to a thorough way to deal with respiratory prosperity.

Ordinary Actual work as a Melodic Development: Integrate customary actual work into your way of life. Practice upgrades cardiovascular wellbeing as well as adds to by and large respiratory capability. The melodic development of actual work supplements the omega-3 ensemble, advancing an agreeable interchange of wellbeing advancing variables.

Sufficient Hydration for Fluidic Agreement: Guarantee satisfactory hydration to keep up with the fluidic balance in the respiratory framework. Hydration upholds the mucous films in the aviation routes, working with ideal respiratory capability. As you appreciate the omega-3 orchestra with salmon, let the fluidic concordance of hydration enhance its resonances.

Quality Rest as a Musical Hold back: Focus on quality rest to help respiratory and generally wellbeing. Rest assumes a significant part in the body's maintenance and upkeep processes, adding to the musical refrain of prosperity. As salmon's omega-3 tune resonates through your dietary decisions, let the helpful notes of value rest enhance its effect.

Stress The executives for Amicable Wellbeing: Carry out pressure the board practices to make an agreeable background for respiratory prosperity. Constant pressure can adversely influence lung capability, and procedures like care, reflection, and unwinding methods structure a contradiction to the omega-3 ensemble, cultivating a condition of adjusted wellbeing.

Tobacco Evasion for Continuous Harmonies: Keep away from tobacco smoke and focus on a without smoke climate. Tobacco smoke is a significant respiratory aggravation, disturbing the harmonies of respiratory wellbeing. As you enjoy the dietary rhythm of salmon's omega-3s, let the continuous harmonies stretch out to a sans tobacco way of life.

Natural Contemplations for Air Quality Affirmation: Be aware of ecological elements that might influence air quality. Guaranteeing great indoor air quality and limiting openness to poisons add to the musical reverberation of respiratory wellbeing. The omega-3 aria of salmon finds full articulation in a climate encourages perfect and empowering air.

Ordinary Wellbeing Exams for Preventive Crescendos: Focus on normal wellbeing tests to screen respiratory wellbeing and address any arising concerns proactively. Preventive medical services turns into a crescendo in the orchestra of prosperity, considering convenient mediations and changes in accordance with keep up with ideal respiratory capability.

Culinary Imagination and Wholesome Insight: Embracing the Orchestra of Respiratory Prosperity

In the orchestra of respiratory prosperity, where the omega-3 aria of salmon becomes the dominant focal point, culinary imagination and wholesome insight become directing notes. Embracing the ensemble includes a powerful interchange of delightful culinary decisions, way of life contemplations, and a profound appreciation for the comprehensive idea of wellbeing.

As you set out on this nourishing excursion, let the omega-3 orchestra of salmon resound through your dinners, bringing scrumptious flavors as well as a musical congruity that upholds respiratory prosperity. From the calming rhythms of EPA to the primary harmonies of DHA, each chomp turns into a melodic commitment to the coordination of wellbeing.

As culinary devotees, wellbeing cognizant people, and searchers of prosperity join in the enthusiasm for salmon's omega-3 lavishness, the ensemble expands its scope. It turns into a common encounter, a cooperative work to support respiratory wellbeing and commend the dietary virtuoso that is salmon. In this amicable investigation, the culinary stage turns into a stage for embracing the ensemble of respiratory prosperity, each flavorful and restorative note in turn.

3.1 Dive into the omega-3 fatty acids found in salmon

Jump into the Omega-3 Unsaturated fats Saw as in Salmon

In the extensive domain of wholesome investigation, the spotlight frequently falls on unambiguous supplements that assume critical parts in supporting in general wellbeing. Among these, omega-3 unsaturated fats arise as key heroes, and the maritime profundities offer a plentiful source — salmon.

This story jumps into the rich oceans of omega-3 unsaturated fats, investigating their importance, the remarkable organization of salmon, and the multi-layered influence they employ in advancing prosperity.

Exploring the Expanse of Omega-3s: A Dietary Endeavor

Prior to diving into the profundities of salmon's omega-3 creation, it is fundamental to leave on a healthful undertaking to grasp the meaning of these fundamental unsaturated fats. Omega-3s address a class of polyunsaturated fats known for their basic jobs in different physiological capabilities. The three essential kinds of omega-3 unsaturated fats are alpha-linolenic corrosive (ALA), eicosapentaenoic corrosive (EPA), and docosahexaenoic corrosive (DHA).

ALA, found in plant-based sources like flaxseeds and chia seeds, fills in as a forerunner for EPA and DHA. While ALA is important, the genuine wholesome reverberation frequently lies in the long-chain unsaturated fats — EPA and DHA — which are prevalently found in greasy fish like salmon. This marine source turns into a wholesome repository, offering an extraordinary structure that lines up with the complex orchestra of wellbeing.

The Salmon Sonata: Omega-3 Structure and Then some

Salmon, frequently hailed as a healthful force to be reckoned with, becomes the overwhelming focus in the omega-3 sonata. Its organization of EPA and DHA makes it a champion wellspring of these fundamental unsaturated fats. The orchestra starts with EPA, an unsaturated fat famous for its mitigating properties. With regards to by and large wellbeing, irritation is a vital participant, frequently embroiled in ongoing illnesses and conditions going from cardiovascular issues to fiery problems.

Studies propose that the calming impacts of EPA can broaden significant advantages, regulating the body's incendiary reaction. The omega-3 sonata, with salmon as its essential entertainer, turns into a restorative song that resounds through the physiological scene, possibly offering help from irritation related illnesses.

DHA, the second development in the salmon sonata, contributes its own arrangement of harmonies to the dietary piece. Plentiful in the cell films of the cerebrum and retina, DHA assumes a urgent part in mental capability and visual wellbeing. Past these domains, DHA's effect reaches out to cardiovascular wellbeing, where it impacts factors, for example, blood thickening and blood vessel wellbeing.

With regards to respiratory prosperity, DHA's underlying scaffolding becomes critical. Found in the cell layers of the lungs, DHA adds to the ease and dependability of these films. This underlying concordance is key to ideal lung capability, guaranteeing that respiratory surfaces stay adaptable and responsive.

The Respiratory Composition: Salmon's Effect on Lung Wellbeing

As the omega-3 sonata keeps on unfurling, a composition arises with regards to respiratory wellbeing. The lungs, complicated organs key to the respiratory framework, benefit from the omega-3 piece viewed as in salmon. Respiratory circumstances, going from asthma to constant obstructive pneumonic infection (COPD), acquaint a remarkable rhythm with the healthful tune.

Asthma, portrayed via aviation route irritation and bronchoconstriction, presents a mind boggling interchange of fiery go betweens. Salmon's omega-3 creation, especially the mitigating notes of EPA, turns into a remedial song that might impact the organization of elements engaged with asthma pathogenesis. Research proposes that an eating regimen wealthy in omega-3s, for example, that got from greasy fish like salmon, may give defensive impacts, possibly moderating the seriousness of asthma side effects.

COPD, an ever-evolving respiratory condition related with constant bronchitis and emphysema, presents an alternate development in the respiratory composition. In people with COPD, steady irritation in the aviation routes and oxidative pressure add to a progressive decrease in lung capability. Salmon's omega-3 aria, with its mitigating and cell reinforcement rhythm, holds guarantee in tending to the ongoing idea of the sickness.

Studies investigating the job of omega-3s, particularly those obtained from marine beginnings like salmon, propose expected benefits. EPA's mitigating impacts might assist with easing side effects, while DHA's underlying scaffolding becomes essential in keeping up with the trustworthiness of lung films. The respiratory song of salmon's omega-3 structure turns into a remedial tune, blending with customary ways to deal with improve respiratory prosperity.

Underneath the Surface: Omega-3s and the Stomach Lung Hub

The orchestra of omega-3s in salmon stretches out past the surface, venturing into the complex environment of the stomach. The stomach lung pivot, a bidirectional correspondence framework between the gastrointestinal lot and the respiratory framework, adds a layer of intricacy to the melodic exchange of nourishment and wellbeing.

Salmon's omega-3 creation adds to the concordance in this microbial city. The calming impacts of EPA and DHA reverberate through the stomach, affecting the equilibrium of the microbiota. A dysregulated stomach microbiome has been connected to different respiratory circumstances, and the omega-3 orchestra, by advancing a sound stomach climate, by implication upholds respiratory prosperity.

Research investigating the stomach lung pivot recommends that the mitigating and immunomodulatory impacts of omega-3s might stretch out to the respiratory framework by adjusting the stomach microbiome. Salmon's rich omega-3 structure turns into a healthful rhythm that reverberations through this interconnected orchestra, cultivating an agreeable connection between the stomach and the lungs.

The stomach, frequently viewed as a key member in generally wellbeing, turns into a unique director in the omega-3 orchestra. As salmon's fundamental unsaturated fats explore the stomach lung pivot, they add to a comprehensive song of wellbeing that stretches out past individual organ frameworks.

Culinary Imagination: Hoisting the Omega-3 Tune with Salmon

As the omega-3 sonata highlighting salmon proceeds with its resounding excursion, culinary imagination turns into a virtuoso in hoisting the wholesome song. The consideration of salmon in a fluctuated and delightful eating regimen opens roads for imaginative culinary articulation, improving both the gustatory experience and the healthful effect.

Fresh Skin Salmon with Spice injected Quinoa: Raise the omega-3 song by container burning salmon to accomplish a firm skin surface. Match it with spice mixed quinoa for a healthy and tasty dish. The blend offers an ensemble of surfaces and tastes while conveying a supplement rich sythesis.

Barbecued Salmon Tacos with Avocado Salsa: Inject a hint of Mexican energy by making barbecued salmon tacos with a reviving avocado salsa. This culinary creation not just commends the omega-3 wealth of salmon yet in addition presents lively flavors and surfaces. The marriage of barbecued salmon and avocado makes an agreeable troupe that reverberates with both wellbeing and guilty pleasure.

Teriyaki Coated Salmon Bowl with Earthy colored Rice: Transport your taste buds to the Far East with a teriyaki coated salmon bowl. Go with the salmon with supplement thick earthy colored rice, making a reasonable and fulfilling dinner. The teriyaki coat adds a sweet and exquisite note, changing the omega-3 ensemble into a culinary show-stopper.

Lemon-Dill Heated Salmon with Cooked Vegetables: Embrace the exemplary blend of lemon and dill in a prepared salmon dish. Supplement the salmon with a variety of broiled vegetables for an outwardly engaging and healthfully rich gathering. The citrusy splendor of lemon and the herbaceous fragrance of dill improve the omega-3 tune with layers of culinary complexity.

Salmon and Spinach Stuffed Portobello Mushrooms: Investigate the universe of stuffed mushrooms by consolidating salmon and spinach. The gritty notes of portobello mushrooms, combined with the lavishness of salmon and the supplement thickness of spinach, make a culinary crescendo. This dish celebrates omega-3s as well as presents a mixture of flavors and surfaces.

Salmon and Asparagus Material Parcels: Embrace the effortlessness of material parcel cooking by getting ready salmon and asparagus groups. The delicate steam made inside the parcels saves the dampness of the salmon while permitting the flavors to merge. This culinary methodology changes the omega-3 sonata into a fragile and invigorating group.

Hot Cajun Darkened Salmon Plate of mixed greens: Implant a smidgen of zest into your culinary collection with a hot Cajun darkened salmon serving of mixed greens. The strong kinds of Cajun preparing add a powerful note to the omega-3 song, making a dish that tempts the taste buds while conveying a supplement pressed encounter.

Salmon and Quinoa-stuffed Chime Peppers: Consolidate the healthful lavishness of salmon and quinoa in a brilliant troupe by getting ready stuffed ringer peppers. This culinary creation not just features the omega-3 structure of salmon yet additionally presents different healthy fixings. The dynamic tones and flavors make this dish an ensemble of wellbeing and gastronomic joy.

Healthful Insight: Past Culinary Imagination

While culinary imagination becomes the overwhelming focus in praising the omega-3 ensemble of salmon, wholesome insight envelops more extensive contemplations that add to in general prosperity. Past the kitchen, way of life decisions, natural variables, and a nuanced comprehension of individual healthful requirements become fundamental parts of the musical experience.

Customary Actual work as an Integral Development: Match the omega-3 sonata with normal active work. Practice upgrades cardiovascular wellbeing as well as adds to generally speaking respiratory capability. The cadenced development of active work turns into a correlative dance in the ensemble of wellbeing, enhancing the advantages of omega-3s saw as in salmon.

Careful Hydration for Fluidic Agreement: Orchestrate the omega-3 song with careful hydration. Sufficient water admission upholds the fluidic balance in the respiratory framework, guaranteeing ideal mucous layer capability. As you enjoy the healthful rhythm of salmon's omega-3s, let the fluidic amicability of hydration intensify its resonances.

Quality Rest as a Helpful Development: Focus on quality rest to help the supportive developments of the omega-3 orchestra. Rest assumes a significant part in the body's maintenance processes, adding to generally prosperity. The supportive notes of value rest become a fundamental development in the ensemble of wellbeing, fitting with the omega-3 rhythm.

Stress The executives for Agreeable Wellbeing: Consolidate pressure the board practices to make an amicable scenery for prosperity. Ongoing pressure can adversely influence lung capability, and systems like care, reflection, and unwinding methods structure a contrast to the omega-3 ensemble, encouraging a condition of adjusted wellbeing.

Tobacco Evasion for Continuous Harmonies: Develop a without tobacco way of life to guarantee continuous harmonies in the ensemble of respiratory wellbeing. Tobacco smoke is a significant respiratory aggravation, upsetting the harmonies of prosperity. As you enjoy the omega-3 tune, let the continuous harmonies reach out to a without smoke climate.

Ecological Contemplations for Clean Air Reverberation: Be aware of natural factors that might influence air quality. Guaranteeing great indoor air quality and limiting openness to poisons add to the musical reverberation of respiratory wellbeing. The omega-3 aria of salmon finds full articulation in a climate encourages perfect and energizing air.

Customary Wellbeing Tests for Preventive Crescendos: Focus on normal wellbeing exams to screen respiratory wellbeing and address any arising concerns proactively. Preventive medical care turns into a crescendo in the ensemble of prosperity, considering ideal mediations and changes in accordance with keep up with ideal respiratory capability.

Culinary Inventiveness and Wholesome Insight: Embracing the Orchestra of Omega-3s

In the fantastic orchestra of sustenance, where every supplement adds to the general wellbeing sythesis, the omega-3 sonata highlighting salmon turns into a show-stopper. The exchange of EPA and DHA, the calming rhythm, the primary harmonies, and the expected commitments to conditions going from asthma to respiratory prosperity paint a rich embroidery of dietary congruity.

As people explore the oceans of culinary inventiveness and dietary insight, the consideration of salmon turns into an intentional and wellbeing cognizant choice — a decision to embrace the omega-3 orchestra and permit its resonances to reverberate through the halls of prosperity. From the culinary happiness regarding imaginative dishes to the nuanced interaction of supplements and the more extensive contemplations of way of life decisions, the omega-3 sonata including salmon turns out to be in excess of a dinner — it turns into a festival of wellbeing, a song that orchestrates with the rhythms of prosperity.

In this agreeable investigation, the culinary stage turns into a stage for embracing the orchestra of omega-3s — each heavenly and energizing note in turn. As the omega-3 sonata keeps on unfurling, it welcomes people to participate in the festival of healthful lavishness, culinary imagination, and the comprehensive reverberation of prosperity. In the continuous story of wellbeing, the omega-3 sonata highlighting salmon stands as an immortal song — a dietary magnum opus that resounds through the oceans of sustenance and the orchestra of life.

Orchestrating Healthful Insight with Omega-3 Dominance: A More profound Plunge into Salmon's Effect on Prosperity

As we plunge further into the expanse of dietary insight and the dominance of omega-3s viewed as in salmon, it is basic to investigate extra features that add to comprehensive prosperity. Past the culinary imagination and way of life contemplations, let us unwind the embroidered artwork of omega-3 dominance and its expected effect on unambiguous medical issue, dive into feasible obtaining rehearses, and investigate the crossing point of omega-3s with arising research in the field of nutrigenomics.

Designated Harmonies: Omega-3s and Cardiovascular Flexibility

While the omega-3 sonata reverberates through different parts of wellbeing, its effect on cardiovascular strength merits unique consideration. The heart, an essential orchestrator in the ensemble of prosperity, benefits from the calming and cardiovascular-defensive properties of omega-3 unsaturated fats, especially EPA and DHA.

Studies have recommended that integrating omega-3-rich food sources, like salmon, into the eating regimen might add to cardiovascular wellbeing by diminishing the gamble of cardiovascular occasions, bringing down circulatory strain, and further developing lipid profiles. The omega-3 tune, with salmon as a noticeable soloist, turns into a cardiovascular concerto that blends with way of life decisions to brace the versatility of the heart.

As people set out on their dietary process, the consideration of salmon turns into an essential move — an interest in the cardiovascular ensemble that reverberations through the passageways of heart wellbeing. The harmonies of omega-3s, when woven into the texture of a heart-sound way of life, make a full creation that addresses the getting through nature of prosperity.

Ecological Concordance: Obtaining Salmon Economically

As we explore the nourishing oceans, the significance of natural contemplations turns into an essential development in the orchestra of prosperity. Feasible obtaining rehearses for salmon line up with moral and biological standards, guaranteeing that the omega-3 tune isn't to the detriment of natural concordance.

Wild-got salmon, obtained through feasible fishing rehearses, frequently conveys a better omega-3 profile contrasted with its ranch raised partners. Selecting wild-got salmon adds to the conservation of marine biological systems, advances dependable fisheries the executives, and guarantees the continuous accessibility of this nourishing virtuoso.

The omega-3 sonata, when acted working together with supportable obtaining rehearses, turns into a tune that reverberates with a more extensive ethos of natural stewardship. It mirrors a pledge to the sensitive equilibrium of nature, recognizing that the soundness of the planet is unpredictably connected to the strength of its occupants.

Congruity in the Genomic Scene: Omega-3s and Nutrigenomics

The convergence of omega-3s with the arising field of nutrigenomics adds a layer of complexity to the healthful orchestra. Nutrigenomics investigates the complicated interaction between dietary parts and quality articulation, offering experiences into how supplements, including omega-3 unsaturated fats, can regulate the hereditary scene.

Research in nutrigenomics recommends that omega-3s might apply their useful impacts by affecting quality articulation connected with aggravation, lipid digestion, and cardiovascular capability. The omega-3 sonata, with salmon as its instrumentalist, turns into a unique power that draws in with the hereditary organization of wellbeing.

People with explicit hereditary varieties might answer distinctively to omega-3 supplementation or dietary admission. The customized idea of nutrigenomics accentuates the requirement for custom-made wholesome methodologies, where the omega-3 orchestra can be adjusted to line up with individual hereditary inclinations.

As the field of nutrigenomics unfurls, the omega-3 sonata highlighting salmon turns into a central member in the developing story of customized nourishment. It opens roads for accuracy ways to deal with prosperity, where the wholesome ensemble isn't just valued for its general effect but on the other hand is figured out with regards to individual hereditary subtleties.

Reverberation in Conceptive Wellbeing: Omega-3s and Pregnancy

The omega-3 sonata stretches out its reverberation to the domain of conceptive wellbeing, where the consideration of salmon in the eating regimen assumes a huge part, especially during pregnancy. Omega-3 unsaturated fats, particularly DHA, are urgent for fetal cerebrum and eye advancement.

Research proposes that maternal utilization of omega-3-rich food sources, like salmon, may add to worked on mental results in kids. The omega-3 tune turns into a cradlesong that supports the formative ensemble of the unborn kid, establishing the groundwork for mental prosperity.

Moreover, omega-3s display calming properties that can be helpful during pregnancy by possibly diminishing the gamble of preterm birth and supporting generally speaking maternal wellbeing. The harmonies of omega-3s, when incorporated into pre-birth sustenance, become a song that reverberations through ages, impacting the wellbeing directions of both mother and kid.

An Ensemble of Prosperity with Salmon's Omega-3 Dominance

In the fabulous ensemble of prosperity, the omega-3 sonata highlighting salmon arises as a magnum opus that reverberates through the different scenes of wellbeing. From cardiovascular versatility and ecological congruity to the complexities of nutrigenomics and the supporting notes in conceptive wellbeing, salmon's omega-3 dominance makes an orchestra that rises above the limits of individual wellbeing parts.

As people explore the nourishing oceans, the incorporation of salmon becomes a dietary decision as well as an amicable articulation of prosperity. The omega-3 sonata, with its complex effect, welcomes people to partake in the continuous story of wellbeing — an account that envelops the heart, the climate, the hereditary scene, and the continuum of life.

The culinary imagination that hoists the omega-3 song, the economical obtaining rehearses that line up with ecological amicability, the nuanced comprehension of nutrigenomics, and the reverberation in conceptive wellbeing on the whole add to the ensemble of prosperity. In this musical investigation, salmon's omega-3 dominance turns into an immortal tune — a song that fits with the rhythms of life, reverberating through the passages of wellbeing and leaving a getting through engrave on the story of prosperity.

3.2 Discuss the anti-inflammatory properties and their impact on lung health

The calming properties of different dietary parts, especially those found in specific food varieties like greasy fish, hold critical ramifications for respiratory prosperity, especially with regards to lung wellbeing. Among these dietary components, omega-3 unsaturated fats, overwhelmingly eicosapentaenoic corrosive (EPA) and docosahexaenoic corrosive (DHA), assume an essential part in tweaking fiery reactions inside the body. The complicated ensemble of irritation includes a mind boggling fountain of sub-atomic occasions, and deviations in this cycle can add to the turn of events and compounding of respiratory circumstances like asthma, ongoing obstructive pneumonic sickness (COPD), and even cellular breakdown in the lungs.

As we dive into the mitigating properties of omega-3 unsaturated fats, it's fundamental to comprehend the nuanced interaction among irritation and lung wellbeing. Provocative cycles are a characteristic and defensive reaction of the body to destructive upgrades, like diseases or wounds. Be that as it may, when aggravation becomes persistent or dysregulated, it can prompt tissue harm and add to the pathogenesis of different respiratory issues.

Omega-3 unsaturated fats, plentifully present in greasy fish like salmon, apply their mitigating impacts through a few systems. EPA, specifically, fills in as a substrate for the development of particular supportive of settling lipid middle people (SPMs, for example, resolvins and protectins. These SPMs effectively advance the goal of aggravation by hosing fiery signals and working with the freedom of incendiary cells. With regards to lung wellbeing, the capacity of omega-3s to advance the goal of irritation is of fundamental significance, as persistent aggravation in the respiratory framework can prompt aviation route rebuilding and hindered lung capability.

Studies have investigated the effect of omega-3 unsaturated fats on unambiguous respiratory circumstances, and asthma stands apart as a remarkable model. Asthma is portrayed by constant aviation route irritation and bronchoconstriction, and the calming properties of omega-3s present in salmon hold guarantee in relieving the seriousness of asthma side effects. Research recommends that an eating regimen wealthy in omega-3 unsaturated fats might diminish the development of supportive of fiery substances, for example, leukotrienes, and improve the creation of mitigating middle people.

In the domain of COPD, a dynamic respiratory condition frequently connected with ongoing bronchitis and emphysema, the calming rhythm of omega-3s turns into a likely partner. COPD includes tenacious irritation in the aviation routes, joined by oxidative pressure, and the capacity of omega-3s to regulate these fiery cycles is a subject of interest in continuous examination. A few examinations have shown that expanded admission of omega-3 unsaturated fats might helpfully affect side effects and lung capability in people with COPD.

Cellular breakdown in the lungs, one more huge worry in the range of respiratory wellbeing, is complicatedly connected to fiery cycles. While omega-3 unsaturated fats are not a remedy for cellular breakdown in the lungs, their mitigating properties might add to a steady climate that supplements regular medicines. Also, continuous exploration is investigating the likely job of omega-3s in regulating the provocative microenvironment inside lung growths, fully intent on impacting illness movement.

The calming orchestra of omega-3s stretches out past the lungs to envelop the stomach lung pivot, a bidirectional correspondence framework between the gastrointestinal lot and the respiratory framework. The stomach microbiota, impacted by the calming impacts of omega-3s, assumes a critical part in molding resistant reactions, and disturbances in stomach microbial equilibrium have been connected to respiratory circumstances. By cultivating a fair and calming stomach climate, omega-3s add to the multifaceted interchange between the stomach and the lungs, by implication supporting respiratory prosperity.

While the emphasis on mitigating properties frequently fixates on omega-3 unsaturated fats, recognizing the more extensive dietary context is urgent. An eating regimen wealthy in natural products, vegetables, and other calming food sources supplements the impacts of omega-3s, making a synergistic group that upholds generally speaking wellbeing, including respiratory prosperity. The Mediterranean eating routine, famous for its mitigating and cardiovascular advantages, consolidates numerous components, like olive oil, natural products, vegetables, and greasy fish, that add to the agreeable ensemble of wellbeing.

As people consider consolidating calming food varieties, remembering salmon rich for omega-3s, into their weight control plans, the more extensive way of life setting turns out to be similarly huge. Customary active work, sufficient hydration, stress the executives, and evasion of tobacco smoke add to the general calming rhythm. Chasing after lung wellbeing, these way of life factors fit with the wholesome orchestra, establishing a climate helpful for respiratory prosperity.

It's critical to take note of that while mitigating food varieties, remembering those rich for omega-3s, offer expected benefits, they are not a panacea. Respiratory wellbeing is an intricate transaction of hereditary, ecological, and way of life factors. Also, individual reactions to dietary mediations might shift. Hence, an all encompassing methodology that incorporates dietary insight with way of life contemplations and, when important, clinical direction is fundamental.

The calming properties of omega-3 unsaturated fats, especially those viewed as in salmon, add to the ensemble of respiratory prosperity. From the complicated balance of provocative reactions in conditions like asthma and COPD to the possible help with regards to cellular breakdown in the lungs, omega-3s assume a multi-layered part. The stomach lung hub, way of life contemplations, and the more extensive dietary setting further enhance the ensemble, establishing an amicable climate that resounds through the passageways of respiratory wellbeing. As people embrace the mitigating tune through careful dietary decisions and comprehensive prosperity rehearses, they leave on an excursion of musical reverberation — one that praises the complicated exchange between nourishment, irritation, and lung wellbeing.

3.3 Tasty salmon-based recipes and meal plans for optimal respiratory support

Setting out on a culinary excursion that tempts the taste buds as well as supports ideal respiratory wellbeing includes the inventive reconciliation of supplement rich fixings, with salmon becoming the overwhelming focus as a dietary virtuoso. Creating a collection of flavorful and energizing recipes, combined with even dinner plans, gives a musical way to deal with respiratory help. From exquisite primary courses to energetic plates of mixed greens and healthy dishes, each dish turns into a culinary note in the amicable troupe of prosperity.

Culinary Suggestion: Barbecued Salmon with Lemon-Dill Quinoa and Cooked Vegetables

Start the gastronomic orchestra with a Barbecued Salmon show-stopper joined by Lemon-Dill Quinoa and Simmered Vegetables. The fresh skin of the barbecued salmon adds a great surface, while the delicious tissue overflows with omega-3 lavishness. The quinoa, imbued with the splendid notes of lemon and the herbaceous fragrance of dill, supplements the salmon's flavor profile. Matched with a vivid variety of simmered vegetables, this dish fulfills the sense of taste as well as conveys a supplement stuffed crescendo that resounds with respiratory prosperity.

Supplement Rich Intermission: Salmon and Spinach Stuffed Portobello Mushrooms

Progress to a supplement rich break with Salmon and Spinach Stuffed Portobello Mushrooms. The hearty notes of the portobello mushrooms give a vigorous scenery to the lavishness of salmon and the supplement thickness of spinach. This culinary organization presents a mixture of flavors and surfaces, making a dish that celebrates omega-3 overflow while offering an ensemble of nutrients and minerals. The stuffed mushrooms, heated flawlessly, become a flavorful note in the culinary collection intended to blend with respiratory help.

Mediterranean Song: Salmon and Feta Salad with Balsamic Vinaigrette

Allow the culinary song to go on with a Mediterranean-propelled salad highlighting Salmon and Feta with a sprinkle of Balsamic Vinaigrette. This lively outfit consolidates the omega-3 lavishness of salmon with the tart notes of feta cheddar. The freshness of new vegetables, enhanced with a balsamic vinaigrette, adds layers of flavor and sustenance.

The ensemble of surfaces, from the flakiness of salmon to the mash of vegetables, makes a plate of mixed greens that charms the faculties as well as adds to the respiratory concordance of prosperity.

Asian Combination Composition: Teriyaki Coated Salmon Bowl with Earthy colored Rice

Mix an Asian combination song into the culinary ensemble with a Teriyaki Coated Salmon Bowl joined by healthy earthy colored rice. The teriyaki coat bestows a sweet and exquisite note to the delicious salmon, making an amicable mix of flavors. Matched with supplement thick earthy colored rice and a beautiful exhibit of vegetables, this bowl turns into a culinary crescendo that joins the omega-3 extravagance of salmon with the healthy integrity of entire grains and vegetables, adding to a balanced respiratory-strong dinner.

Zesty Cajun Congruity: Darkened Salmon Tacos with Avocado Salsa

Investigate a zesty Cajun congruity with Darkened Salmon Tacos highlighting a reviving Avocado Salsa. The strong kinds of Cajun preparing add a unique note to the omega-3 extravagance of darkened salmon. Settled in delicate taco shells and finished off with an energetic avocado salsa, this dish fulfills the zest lovers as well as presents an orchestra of surfaces and tastes. The richness of avocado, the intensity of Cajun flavors, and the flakiness of salmon make a culinary magnum opus that resounds with both extravagance and respiratory help.

Firm Joy: Fresh Skin Salmon with Spice injected Quinoa

Hoist the culinary notes with a Firm Skin Salmon joined by Spice injected Quinoa. The dish singed salmon, with its fresh outside, turns into a visual pleasure while holding the omega-3 wealth inside. The quinoa, imbued with sweet-smelling spices, adds a layer of intricacy to the dish. Matched with a side of steamed vegetables, this creation offers an orchestra of flavors and surfaces that satisfies the sense of taste as well as adds to the wholesome rhythm supporting respiratory wellbeing.

Culinary Combination: Miso-Coated Salmon with Soba Noodle Salad

Set out on a culinary combination venture with Miso-Coated Salmon served close by a Soba Noodle Salad. The umami-rich miso coat upgrades the flavor profile of the delicious salmon, while the soba noodle salad presents a magnificent mixture of surfaces. Supplemented by different new vegetables and an exquisite miso dressing, this dish turns into an agreeable combination of flavors that weds the omega-3 extravagance of salmon with the wonderful components of Japanese food, offering a culinary orchestra for respiratory prosperity.

Veggie lover Two part harmony: Quinoa and Broiled Vegetable Stuffed Chime Peppers

Create a veggie lover two part harmony with Quinoa and Cooked Vegetable Stuffed Ringer Peppers, including the supplement rich decency of quinoa and a bright gathering of broiled vegetables. While salmon takes a short interval, the emphasis stays on a supplement thick structure that lines up with respiratory help.

The dynamic ringer peppers, loaded up with quinoa and broiled vegetables, become a culinary tune that celebrates plant-based sustenance and offers a wonderful respite in the omega-3 orchestra.

Culinary Goal: Lemon-Dill Prepared Salmon with Simmered Asparagus

Close the culinary excursion with a light yet tasty Lemon-Dill Heated Salmon matched with Broiled Asparagus. The effortlessness of baking permits the normal kinds of salmon to sparkle, improved by the citrusy brilliance of lemon and the herbaceous notes of dill. Broiled asparagus, with its delicate freshness, adds a correlative component to the dish. This culinary goal carries the omega-3 ensemble to a delicate close, offering a sense of taste purging yet fulfilling note in the climax of respiratory-accommodating recipes.

Making Respiratory-Strong Dinner Plans: A Healthful Sonata

Past individual culinary pieces, the creating of respiratory-strong feast plans includes coordinating a dietary sonata that traverses breakfast, lunch, and supper. Consolidating various supplement thick food varieties, with an emphasis on those wealthy in omega-3 unsaturated fats, makes an ensemble of flavors and supplements that add to generally speaking respiratory prosperity.

Breakfast Composition: Smoked Salmon and Avocado Toast

Initiate the day with a Morning meal Composition including Smoked Salmon and Avocado Toast. This dish gives a good beginning as well as presents omega-3 lavishness promptly in the day. The mix of smoked salmon, smooth avocado, and entire grain toast makes a reasonable and fulfilling breakfast that lines up with respiratory help.

Noontime Song: Quinoa Salad with Chipped Salmon

Noontime carries a reviving tune with a Quinoa Salad highlighting chipped salmon. The quinoa, threw with various vegetables and spices, turns into a supplement stuffed base, while the chipped salmon adds a protein support. The variety of surfaces and flavors offers a healthy and stimulating note in the late morning dinner, adding to the generally nourishing ensemble.

Evening Interval: Greek Yogurt Parfait with Berries and Pecans

Make a midday recess with a Greek Yogurt Parfait enhanced with berries and pecans. Greek yogurt gives a protein-rich establishment, while the berries contribute cell reinforcements. The omega-3 extravagance of pecans adds a superb crunch and dietary profundity to the parfait. This light yet feeding break turns into a sweet note in the respiratory-strong feast plan.

Supper Finale: Prepared Salmon with Yam and Broccoli

Finish up the day's healthful orchestra with a Supper Finale including Prepared Salmon joined by yams and broccoli. The heated salmon, with its straightforwardness and omega-3 lavishness, becomes the overwhelming focus.

Yams, plentiful in nutrients and fiber, and broccoli, a cruciferous vegetable, add to the nourishing crescendo. This supper finale offers an amicable mix of flavors and supplements that line up with ideal respiratory help.

A Nourishing Coda: Embracing Assortment and Control

As people leave on an excursion of creating respiratory-steady feast designs, embracing assortment and moderation is critical. Consolidating a different scope of supplement thick food varieties guarantees an orchestra of nutrients, minerals, and cell reinforcements, adding to generally speaking prosperity. While salmon plays an unmistakable job in giving omega-3 unsaturated fats, an offset with other protein sources, entire grains, organic products, and vegetables makes a nourishing coda that reverberates with all encompassing wellbeing.

Moreover, balance in segment sizes and careful eating rehearses adds a nuanced layer to the wholesome ensemble. Focusing on craving and completion prompts, relishing each chomp, and developing a careful way to deal with dinners add to the general delight and viability of a respiratory-strong feast plan.

Culinary Innovativeness and Prosperity: A Supported Tune

In the fabulous organization of culinary imagination and prosperity, the supported tune of respiratory help is woven into the texture of every recipe and feast plan. From the flavorful notes of barbecued salmon to the reviving intervals of plates of mixed greens and the encouraging goals of prepared dishes, the culinary ensemble turns into a festival of wellbeing and gastronomic joy.

As people investigate the different creations and nourishing sonatas, they leave on an excursion that reaches out past the joy of eating to the significant effect on respiratory prosperity. The omega-3 extravagance of salmon, supplemented by an orchestra of supplement thick food sources, turns into a dietary rhythm that reverberates through the passageways of ideal wellbeing.

In this culinary investigation, the kitchen turns into an imaginative stage, and every dinner is a potential chance to add to the continuous orchestra of prosperity. The transaction of flavors, surfaces, and dietary parts fits with the more extensive way of life contemplations, making a supported song that celebrates respiratory wellbeing and the delight of feeding the body with tasty and stimulating manifestations. As people embrace the culinary imagination and prosperity rehearses, they become members in a supported and amicable song — a tune that praises the multifaceted exchange between sustenance, culinary imaginativeness, and the orchestra of life.

Musical Eating: Salmon Nibbles with Herbed Yogurt Plunge

Lift eating to a musical involvement in Salmon Chomps matched with a Herbed Yogurt Plunge. These reduced down delights highlight chipped salmon, bound along with spices and a dash of breadcrumbs, making flavorful pieces wealthy in omega-3 goodness.

The herbed yogurt plunge, imbued with new dill, adds an invigorating and tart note to each nibble. This nibble fulfills desires as well as presents a great interval of respiratory help, making it an ideal backup to the culinary ensemble.

Debauched Sweet Coda: Dim Chocolate-Plunged Salmon Chomps

Finish up the culinary excursion with a wanton treat coda — Dull Chocolate-Plunged Salmon Chomps. This startling yet amicable matching joins the rich kinds of dull chocolate with the flakiness of salmon. The omega-3 wealth of salmon finds a sweet partner in the cell reinforcements present in dim chocolate. This liberal treat satisfies sweet desires as well as adds an interesting and critical note to the culinary collection, making a wonderful end to the ensemble of salmon-based recipes.

Wholesome Crescendo: Grasping the Advantages

Past the culinary joy and gastronomic innovativeness, it's fundamental to comprehend the healthful crescendo that these salmon-based recipes add to respiratory prosperity. Salmon, a greasy fish wealthy in omega-3 unsaturated fats, offers a scope of medical advantages, especially with regards to lung wellbeing.

Omega-3 Extravagance: Salmon stands as a force to be reckoned with of omega-3 unsaturated fats, especially EPA and DHA. These fundamental unsaturated fats assume a critical part in regulating irritation, supporting cardiovascular wellbeing, and adding to generally speaking prosperity. The omega-3 wealth of salmon turns into a dietary foundation in the orchestra of respiratory help.

Mitigating Properties: The calming rhythm of omega-3 unsaturated fats lines up with the intricate exchange of aggravation and lung wellbeing. By advancing the goal of irritation, omega-3s add to a decent resistant reaction and may have valuable impacts in respiratory circumstances portrayed by constant irritation.

Protein Ability: Salmon is a great wellspring of protein, giving fundamental amino acids that add to the maintenance and support of tissues. Protein is a major structure block for respiratory wellbeing, supporting the construction and capability of muscles engaged with relaxing.

Wealthy in Supplements: notwithstanding omega-3s and protein, salmon is plentiful in different supplements, including vitamin D, vitamin B12, selenium, and iodine. These supplements assume different parts in generally wellbeing, including safe capability, energy digestion, and thyroid wellbeing, all of which add to respiratory prosperity.

Various Culinary Supplements: The culinary ensemble stretches out past salmon to incorporate a different cluster of supplement thick fixings. From the cell reinforcement rich vegetables to the fiber-stuffed quinoa and the probiotic decency of yogurt, every part adds layers of wholesome profundity to the general creation.

Careful Culinary Practices: The culinary excursion itself turns into a training in care, underscoring the significance of relishing each chomp, appreciating the flavors, and developing a positive relationship with food. Careful eating adds to by and large prosperity, cultivating a comprehensive methodology that reaches out past nourishing substance.

As people participate in the culinary ensemble of salmon-based recipes, they appreciate scrumptious dinners as well as effectively take part in the organization of their wellbeing. The wholesome wealth, calming properties, and culinary inventiveness woven into these recipes make a supported song that reverberates through the halls of respiratory prosperity.

A Culinary Festival of Respiratory Wellbeing

In the excellent culinary festival of respiratory wellbeing, salmon arises as the star entertainer, contributing its omega-3 wealth, calming properties, and culinary flexibility to the ensemble of prosperity. From exquisite primary courses to reviving plates of mixed greens, reduced down tidbits, and, surprisingly, liberal treats, every recipe turns into a note in the agreeable creation that upholds ideal lung wellbeing.

As people leave on this culinary excursion, they feed their bodies as well as take part in a festival of the faculties. The energetic varieties, various surfaces, and rich kinds of these salmon-based manifestations make a multisensory experience that reaches out past nourishment to the domain of gastronomic euphoria.

The orchestra of salmon-based recipes welcomes people to embrace a way of life where culinary innovativeness and respiratory prosperity merge. It supports careful eating, dietary insight, and a nuanced comprehension of the interaction among food and wellbeing. In the continuous story of prosperity, the culinary festival of respiratory wellbeing turns into an immortal tune — a song that blends with the rhythms of life and reverberations through the hallways of all encompassing wellbeing.

Chapter 4

Kale Crescendo
Vitamins Fortify Respiratory Strength

Collecting Respiratory Flexibility: The Kale Crescendo

In the ensemble of nourishing insight, kale arises as a virtuoso, a verdant green stalwart that coordinates a crescendo of nutrients to sustain respiratory strength. As an individual from the cruciferous vegetable family, kale not just adds to the liveliness of culinary manifestations yet in addition winds around a wholesome embroidery that reverberates with the mind boggling requirements of the respiratory framework. Allow us to set out on an excursion through the kale crescendo, investigating the different nutrients it brings to the front and their significant effect on respiratory strength.

Vitamin A: Enlightening Lung Wellbeing

At the front of the kale crescendo is Vitamin A, a central member in enlightening lung wellbeing. This fundamental nutrient is essential to the support of respiratory epithelial cells, adding to the honesty of the mucosal covering in the lungs.

As a powerful cell reinforcement, Vitamin A battles oxidative pressure, an element connected to the turn of events and movement of respiratory circumstances. Kale, with its lively green tints, implies the presence of beta-carotene, a forerunner to Vitamin A, making it a healthful foundation in encouraging respiratory strength.

L-ascorbic acid: The Safeguard Against Oxidative Orchestra

As the kale crescendo arrives at its pinnacle, L-ascorbic acid becomes the overwhelming focus — an impressive safeguard against the oxidative ensemble that can think twice about prosperity. Kale, with its liberal L-ascorbic acid substance, turns into a gatekeeper of lung wellbeing by killing free revolutionaries and reinforcing the body's cell reinforcement protections. This water-solvent nutrient assumes an essential part in collagen combination, adding to the primary trustworthiness of lung tissues. Through its mitigating properties, L-ascorbic acid coordinates an agreeable equilibrium inside the respiratory framework, making a defensive song against oxidative pressure.

Vitamin K: Planning Hemostasis and Aggravation

In the kale crescendo, Vitamin K takes on an unpretentious yet critical job, planning hemostasis and irritation inside the respiratory scene. This fat-dissolvable nutrient, richly present in kale, partakes in the combination of proteins associated with blood coagulating and aggravation guideline. By encouraging a fragile equilibrium, Vitamin K adds to the counteraction of unnecessary irritation, a variable embroiled in the pathogenesis of respiratory issues. The kale crescendo, with its Vitamin K wealth, consequently turns into a nuanced structure that upholds both respiratory and circulatory prosperity.

Vitamin B6: Supporting Synapses for Respiratory Agreement

The kale crescendo keeps on unfurling with the consideration of Vitamin B6, a supplement that plays a supporting job in the combination of synapses. Past its old style relationship with energy digestion, Vitamin B6 adds to the development of serotonin and dopamine, synapses with modulatory impacts on respiratory control communities. In the kale orchestra, Vitamin B6 turns into an unpretentious yet critical note, cultivating a brain climate helpful for respiratory concordance.

Vitamin E: Cancer prevention agent Virtuosity in Respiratory Safeguard

As the kale crescendo spreads out, Vitamin E ventures onto the stage, displaying its cell reinforcement virtuosity in respiratory guard. This fat-dissolvable nutrient, tracked down in kale in striking sums, fills in as a safeguard against oxidative harm to cell films. In the respiratory scene, where openness to natural poisons is unavoidable, Vitamin E turns into a safeguard of lung cell trustworthiness. By killing free revolutionaries, Vitamin E adds to the general cancer prevention agent orchestra that sustains respiratory strength.

Folate: Arranging DNA Blend for Cell Congruity

Folate, an individual from the B-nutrient family, assumes a crucial part in the kale crescendo by organizing DNA union for cell concordance. This nutrient, otherwise called Nutrient B9, is fundamental for the creation and fix of DNA — an essential cycle for the expansion and support of cells, remembering those for the respiratory epithelium. Kale, with its folate overflow, turns into a wellspring of cell support, adding to the recovery and upkeep of tissues fundamental for respiratory capability.

Niacin (Vitamin B3): Empowering Cell Energy for Respiratory Life

In the kale crescendo, Niacin assumes the job of an energy empowering agent, giving the phone fuel important to respiratory force. This B-nutrient, otherwise called Vitamin B3, partakes in the change of food into energy through its contribution in metabolic pathways. By working with the creation of cell energy, Niacin guarantees that the respiratory muscles have the imperative endurance for ideal working. In the kale orchestra, Niacin turns into a note of essentialness that resounds through the passageways of respiratory strength.

Riboflavin (Vitamin B2): Working with Oxygen Use

The kale crescendo arrives at a powerful top with the consideration of Riboflavin, otherwise called Vitamin B2, which assumes a pivotal part in working with oxygen usage. As a part of the electron transport chain, Riboflavin adds to the creation of adenosine triphosphate (ATP), the cell money of energy. With regards to respiratory wellbeing, proficient oxygen use is fundamental, and Riboflavin, tracked down richly in kale, turns into a facilitator of this crucial cycle.

Thiamine (Vitamin B1): Supporting Sensory system Agreement

Finishing the B-nutrient troupe in the kale crescendo is Thiamine, or Vitamin B1, which upholds sensory system amicability. Thiamine is fundamental for the appropriate working of nerve cells and is engaged with the transmission of nerve motivations. In the respiratory ensemble, where brain coordination is central to breathing rhythms, Thiamine turns into a strong note that adds to the consistent exchange of apprehensive signs for ideal respiratory capability.

Mineral Rhythm: Kale's Supplement Ensemble Past Nutrients

Past the ensemble of nutrients, kale adds to respiratory strength through its mineral rhythm. Plentiful in minerals like potassium, magnesium, and calcium, kale upholds the electrolyte balance essential for smooth muscle capability, incorporating the muscles associated with relaxing. Potassium, specifically, assumes a part in keeping up with lung versatility and aviation route patency, further improving the respiratory ensemble directed by kale.

Culinary Suggestion: Integrating Kale into the Tune of Dinners

Integrating kale into the tune of dinners includes a culinary suggestion that commends its wholesome lavishness. From lively plates of mixed greens to exquisite sautés and sustaining smoothies, kale can be a flexible virtuoso in the kitchen.

A Kale and Quinoa Salad, highlighting a mixture of bright vegetables and a lively dressing, turns into a reviving note in the dietary orchestra. A Kale and White Bean Soup, implanted with sweet-smelling spices and flavors, makes an encouraging tune that reverberates with both flavor and respiratory help. The kale crescendo reaches out to a Kale and Berry Smoothie, where the verdant green consolidates with cell reinforcement rich berries to make an amicable mix that satisfies the sense of taste as well as supports the respiratory scene.

Respiratory Reverberation: Kale's Effect on Lung Wellbeing

The kale crescendo, with its ensemble of nutrients and minerals, resounds with a significant effect on lung wellbeing. The blend of cancer prevention agents, calming properties, and cell support found in kale adds to respiratory versatility. The nutrients inside kale assume complex parts — from supporting the underlying honesty of lung tissues to killing oxidative pressure and cultivating brain coordination for ideal breathing examples. As a supplement rich verdant green, kale turns into a director in the coordination of lung wellbeing, making a supported song that reverberations through the halls of respiratory prosperity.

Comprehensive Concordance: Incorporating Kale into a Respiratory-Strong Way of life

The kale crescendo reaches out past the plate to include an all encompassing concordance that incorporates kale into a respiratory-strong way of life. Normal actual work, stress the board, and evasion of tobacco smoke supplement the dietary extravagance of kale, making a synergistic gathering that reverberates with in general prosperity. Embracing kale as a culinary virtuoso turns into a careful decision — one that lines up with the standards of nourishing insight and the quest for an orchestra of wellbeing that incorporates respiratory strength.

Culinary Investigation and Health Orchestra

In the great story of culinary investigation and health, kale remains as a central member in the orchestra of sustenance. Its rich embroidery of nutrients, minerals, and phytonutrients makes an amicable mix that charms the taste buds as well as braces the body, particularly the mind boggling scene of the respiratory framework. The kale crescendo turns into a festival of culinary inventiveness and dietary insight, welcoming people to embrace a way of life where the ensemble of wellbeing unfurls through careful decisions and energetic, sustaining feasts.

As people leave on the excursion of coordinating kale into their culinary collection, they take part in a health orchestra — an ensemble that recognizes the significant effect of sustenance on respiratory versatility and generally essentialness. From the primary chomp of a kale-implanted salad to the last taste of a supplement stuffed smoothie, each culinary note adds to the supported tune of prosperity. In the kale crescendo, people find a culinary virtuoso as well as a nourishing partner — a verdant green that resounds with the ensemble of wellbeing, making a comprehensive concordance that reverberations through the passageways of respiratory strength and then some.

4.1 Explore the nutritional powerhouse of kale and its rich vitamin content

Kale Uncovered: The Dietary Embroidered artwork

In the domain of mixed greens, kale arises as a dietary force to be reckoned with, winding around a rich embroidery of nutrients that add to all encompassing prosperity. As a cruciferous vegetable, kale flaunts a strong flavor as well as conveys an ensemble of fundamental supplements, making it a culinary virtuoso and a healthful partner. Allow us to leave on an excursion to investigate the kaleidoscope of nutrients inside kale, unwinding its wholesome complexities and the significant effect it has on wellbeing.

Vitamin A: The Visionary Gatekeeper

At the front of kale's dietary ability is Vitamin A, a visionary gatekeeper of different physiological capabilities. In kale, Vitamin An appears as beta-carotene, a powerful cell reinforcement that not just confers the dynamic green tone to the leaves yet in addition holds the way to visual wellbeing. As a forerunner to retinol, Vitamin An assumes a urgent part in keeping up with the trustworthiness of the mucous layers, remembering those for the eyes. Its cell reinforcement properties reach out past vision, adding to a strong resistant framework and skin wellbeing. In the kale embroidery, Vitamin A turns into a primary note, reverberating with the ensemble of generally prosperity.

L-ascorbic acid: The Safeguard Against Oxidative Invasion

As the wholesome investigation develops, L-ascorbic acid arises as a safeguard against the oxidative surge that the body faces day to day. Kale's liberal substance of L-ascorbic acid positions it as an impressive protector against free revolutionaries, unsteady particles that can cause cell harm. Past its notable job in safe help, L-ascorbic acid adds to collagen blend, encouraging the wellbeing and flexibility of connective tissues. In the kale embroidery, L-ascorbic acid turns into a defensive note, bracing the body against oxidative pressure and adding to the orchestra of skin wellbeing and safe imperativeness.

Vitamin K: The Guide of Coagulation and Bone Wellbeing

Diving further into kale's dietary creation, Vitamin K becomes the overwhelming focus, organizing coagulation and bone wellbeing. Vitamin K exists in two essential structures — K1 and K2 — and kale conveys a remarkable portion of both. K1, fundamental for blood thickening, guarantees appropriate coagulation and wound recuperating. K2, then again, adds to bone wellbeing by directing calcium affidavit during the bones and veins. In the kale embroidery, Vitamin K turns into a guide of fundamental physiological cycles, orchestrating the sensitive harmony among coagulation and bone honesty.

Vitamin B6: Sustaining Synapses and Digestion

The kale story stretches out to Vitamin B6, a supplement that plays a sustaining job in the union of synapses. This B-nutrient, otherwise called pyridoxine, partakes in the transformation of amino acids, supporting the development of serotonin, dopamine, and different synapses. Past its job in brain wellbeing, Vitamin B6 adds to digestion by supporting the breakdown of sugars, proteins, and fats. In the kale embroidery, Vitamin B6 turns into an unpretentious yet huge note, cultivating a brain climate helpful for state of mind guideline and ideal digestion.

Vitamin E: Cancer prevention agent Guardianship in Cell Protection

In the midst of kale's dietary outfit, Vitamin E arises as a cancer prevention agent gatekeeper, effectively took part in cell protection. This fat-dissolvable nutrient, with its tocopherol variations, fills in as a defender against oxidative pressure by killing free extremists. In doing as such, Vitamin E adds to the safeguarding of cell layer trustworthiness. Its cancer prevention agent virtuosity stretches out to insusceptible help and skin wellbeing, making it a vital piece of the kale embroidery — a note that resounds with the cell guard orchestra.

Folate: The Engineer of DNA Combination and Cell Expansion

As the kale investigation extends, folate assumes the job of a designer, regulating DNA amalgamation and cell expansion. Folate, or Nutrient B9, is essential for the creation and fix of DNA, a key interaction for cell division and tissue development.

Satisfactory folate levels are particularly pivotal during times of fast cell division, like pregnancy. In the kale embroidery, folate turns into a fundamental note, adding to the cell engineering that underlies by and large development, advancement, and support.

Niacin (Vitamin B3): Catalyzing Cell Energy Creation

The kale story reaches out to Niacin, otherwise called Vitamin B3, which catalyzes cell energy creation, a crucial cycle for generally imperativeness. Niacin takes part in the transformation of food into energy through its contribution in metabolic pathways, like glycolysis and the citrus extract cycle. In the kale embroidery, Niacin turns into a note of essentialness, supporting the cell processes that fuel the body's energy needs and add to metabolic concordance.

Riboflavin (Vitamin B2): Encouraging Cell Breath and Development

In the kale crescendo, Riboflavin, or Vitamin B2, ventures onto the stage, encouraging cell breath and development. Riboflavin assumes a significant part in the electron transport chain, a progression of cycles that produce cell energy as adenosine triphosphate (ATP). Past its association in energy creation, Riboflavin adds to cell development and fix. In the kale embroidery, Riboflavin turns into a facilitator of cell essentialness — a note that reverberates with the powerful cycles hidden development and energy digestion.

Thiamine (Vitamin B1): Fundamental Help for Sensory system Capability

Finishing the B-nutrient group in kale is Thiamine, or Vitamin B1, offering fundamental help for sensory system capability. Thiamine is essential to the transmission of nerve motivations and the union of synapses.

In the kale embroidery, Thiamine turns into a strong note, adding to the consistent exchange of apprehensive signs that control different physiological cycles, including muscle constriction and unwinding.

Mineral Rhythm: Past Nutrients, Kale's Mineral Ensemble

Past the ensemble of nutrients, kale adds to dietary concordance through its mineral rhythm. Plentiful in minerals like potassium, magnesium, and calcium, kale upholds different physiological capabilities. Potassium, specifically, assumes a significant part in keeping up with legitimate liquid equilibrium, supporting heart wellbeing, and adding to the general electrolyte concordance important for cell and strong capability. The mineral orchestra in kale supplements its nutrient lavishness, making an extensive nourishing piece that resounds with comprehensive prosperity.

Culinary Ensemble: Kale's Adaptability in the Kitchen

Past its dietary virtuosity, kale's flexibility in the kitchen adds a unique aspect to its culinary ensemble. From dynamic servings of mixed greens to supporting soups and healthy smoothies, kale adjusts to different culinary sytheses, improving both flavor and wholesome thickness. A Kale and Quinoa Salad, enhanced with bright vegetables and a tart dressing, turns into a reviving note in the kale ensemble — a variety of surfaces and tastes that celebrate both culinary imagination and healthful insight. A Kale and White Bean Soup, mixed with fragrant spices and flavors, makes an encouraging tune that reverberates with warmth and sustenance. The kale embroidery stretches out to a Kale and Berry Smoothie, where the verdant green orchestrates with cell reinforcement rich berries, making a dynamic mix that satisfies the sense of taste as well as sustains the body.

All encompassing Concordance: Incorporating Kale into a Decent Way of life

The kale story stretches out past individual supplements and culinary manifestations to include all encompassing congruity — an incorporation of kale into a fair way of life. Actual work, stress the executives, and sufficient rest supplement kale's dietary lavishness, making a synergistic gathering that reverberates with by and large prosperity. Embracing kale as a culinary and dietary partner turns into a careful decision — one that lines up with the standards of adjusted living and the quest for an orchestra of wellbeing that includes physical, mental, and profound imperativeness.

Reverberating Wellbeing: The Kale Ensemble in Wellbeing

In the fantastic story of wellbeing, the kale ensemble reverberates with a significant effect on wellbeing. The kaleidoscope of nutrients, minerals, and phytonutrients inside kale adds to an ensemble of advantages — from supporting resistant capability and cell protection to cultivating brain wellbeing and energy digestion. As people coordinate kale into their culinary collection and way of life, they effectively take part in the organization of their wellbeing, making a supported song that reverberations through the hallways of prosperity.

Culinary Innovativeness: Hoisting the Kale Orchestra

In the domain of culinary innovativeness, kale fills in as a flexible material, welcoming people to hoist the kale orchestra with creative and feeding arrangements. From dynamic servings of mixed greens to exquisite entrées and innovative bites, kale's versatility permits it to orchestrate with different flavors and surfaces. We should investigate how culinary imagination can additionally enhance the kale experience, changing it into a culinary work of art that enchants the taste buds as well as boosts healthful advantages.

Kale Salad Event: A Material of Varieties and Surfaces

One of the quintessential articulations of kale in culinary imaginativeness is the kale salad spectacle — a material of varieties and surfaces that commends the verdant green's vigorous flavor and dietary wealth. Start with a base of new kale leaves, kneading them delicately to upgrade delicacy and decrease harshness. Integrate a variety of dynamic vegetables, for example, cherry tomatoes, chime peppers, and carrots for an eruption of variety and a mixture of nutrients. To add a layer of crunch, incorporate nuts or seeds like almonds or sunflower seeds.

For a hint of smoothness, consider integrating avocado cuts or disintegrated feta cheddar. Lift the flavor profile with a lively dressing, joining olive oil, lemon juice, garlic, and a sprinkle of honey. The outcome is a kale salad party that tempts the taste buds as well as offers an ensemble of nutrients, minerals, and cell reinforcements. This culinary creation turns into a visual and gustatory joy — a kale magnum opus that mirrors the imaginativeness of healthy eating.

Exquisite Kale Entrées: From Sautéed Pleasures to Delightful Sautés

Kale's flexibility reaches out past servings of mixed greens to exquisite entrées that grandstand its capacity to ingest enhances and contribute a good surface. Sautéed kale with garlic and olive oil is a basic yet delightful readiness that emphasizes the verdant green's normal taste. Add a smidgen of stew chips for a sprinkle of intensity, making a powerful dish that matches well with different protein sources like barbecued chicken or tofu.

Integrate kale into sautés, consolidating it with a collection of bright vegetables, lean proteins, and fragrant flavors. The kale's strength and capacity to hold its design make it an optimal expansion to sautés, contributing a healthful lift to the general piece. Whether collapsed into a quinoa pan sear or highlighted in a vegetable variety with earthy colored rice, kale turns into a flavorful note that hoists the healthful profile of the whole dish.

Inventive Kale Tidbits: From Firm Chips to Tasty Pesto

Raise eating with inventive kale manifestations, changing the verdant green into firm chips or a delightful pesto. Kale chips are a famous and nutritious option in contrast to customary potato chips. Just throw kale leaves with olive oil, sprinkle with flavors of decision, and heat until fresh. The outcome is a crunchy bite that furnishes the fulfillment of chip extravagance with the additional advantages of kale's nutrients and minerals.

Kale pesto offers a one of a kind contort on the exemplary basil-based variant. Mix new kale leaves with garlic, pine nuts, Parmesan cheddar, and olive oil to make a lively and supplement thick pesto. Use it as a tasty spread on entire grain wafers or as a pasta sauce for a dish that fits wellbeing and culinary development. These kale-imbued snacks become awesome breaks in the culinary ensemble, demonstrating that healthy eating can be both creative and fulfilling.

Kale Smoothie Polish: Mixing Supplements with Invigorating Flavors

Enter the domain of kale smoothie polish, where the verdant green mixes flawlessly with a variety of products of the soil to make an invigorating and supplement stuffed refreshment. Begin with a base of kale leaves, guaranteeing their stems are eliminated to upgrade perfection. Add a variety of natural products like bananas, berries, and mango for pleasantness and an explosion of cell reinforcements. Integrate a fluid part like almond milk or coconut water to accomplish the ideal consistency.

To upgrade the nourishing profile, present superfoods like chia seeds, flaxseeds, or a scoop of protein powder. The outcome is a kale smoothie that not just fortifies the faculties with its energetic tones yet in addition gives an orchestra of nutrients, minerals, and plant-based supplements. This kale-mixed refreshment turns into a sustaining and hydrating note in the culinary collection — a demonstration of the consistent joining of kale into the universe of refreshingly nutritious beverages.

Culinary Combination: Kale in Worldwide Cooking

Investigate the worldwide impact of kale by integrating it into global cooking styles, where its flexibility and wholesome extravagance can be commended in assorted culinary customs. In Italian cooking, kale can be highlighted in a Tuscan-roused soup with white beans and tomatoes, adding a good and supplement thick component to the dish. In Asian pan-sears, kale flawlessly mixes with soy sauce, ginger, and garlic, offering a healthful lift to conventional flavors.

Embrace Mexican culinary customs by integrating kale into tacos or burritos, consolidating it with lively salsas and delightful flavors. The versatility of kale permits it to consistently coordinate into different worldwide dishes, contributing its healthful orchestra to the worldwide embroidery of culinary variety. This culinary combination exhibits kale's flexibility as well as highlights its true capacity as a staple in kitchens all over the planet.

Culinary Insight: Boosting Wholesome Advantages

As people leave on an excursion of culinary imagination with kale, boosting the nourishing advantages through smart planning and pairings is fundamental. Consider the accompanying culinary insight to improve the wholesome effect of kale-based manifestations:

Balance Flavors and Surfaces: Consolidate kale with various fixings to accomplish an equilibrium between flavors and surfaces. The interchange of sweet, flavorful, crunchy, and smooth components makes a complex culinary encounter.

Match with Reciprocal Fixings: Improve the dietary collaboration by matching kale with fixings that supplement its profile. For instance, L-ascorbic acid rich organic products can improve the ingestion of non-heme iron from kale, streamlining supplement use.

Explore different avenues regarding Flavors: Investigate various flavors and flavors to lift the flavor profile of kale dishes. Spices like basil, thyme, and rosemary can add profundity, while flavors like cumin, turmeric, and paprika contribute warmth and intricacy.

Join with Lean Proteins: Coordinate lean protein sources, like barbecued chicken, tofu, or vegetables, to make balanced and satisfying feasts. The mix of kale's fiber and protein encourages a feeling of totality and fulfillment.

Focus on Entire Food Fixings: Accentuate entire food fixings in kale-based recipes to augment wholesome thickness. Entire grains, nuts, seeds, and brilliant vegetables contribute a variety of nutrients, minerals, and phytonutrients.

Careful Cooking Procedures: Use careful cooking strategies, for example, rubbing kale leaves or gently sautéing them, to improve flavor and delicacy. Careful readiness techniques add to both culinary pleasure and supplement retention.

Culinary Investigation: A Supported Tune of Prosperity

In the fantastic story of culinary investigation, kale remains as a supported song of prosperity — an encouragement to praise the combination of flavor, nourishment, and imagination. From dynamic servings of mixed greens that exhibit kale's newness to exquisite entrées that hoist its goodness, and creative bites that reclassify extravagance, kale's flexibility exceeds all rational limitations.

As people embrace kale in their culinary collection, they participate in an excursion that reaches out past sustenance — it turns into a festival of careful eating, healthful insight, and the delight of enjoying healthy manifestations. Culinary investigation with kale turns into an agreeable exchange of varieties, surfaces, and flavors — an orchestra that resounds with the standards of comprehensive prosperity.

Fundamentally, kale turns out to be in excess of a verdant green; it changes into a culinary sidekick — a supplement rich partner that upgrades the culinary scene while adding to the ensemble of wellbeing. Through each imaginative dish, kale turns into a director in the culinary ensemble, organizing a tune that reverberations through the passageways of comprehensive prosperity — a song that welcomes people to relish the taste, yet the whole experience of healthy eating.

4.2 Practical advice on incorporating kale into daily meals

Orchestrating Wellbeing: Functional Guidance on Integrating Kale into Day to day Dinners

Chasing prosperity, kale arises as a dietary virtuoso, offering an ensemble of nutrients, minerals, and phytonutrients. To tackle the full range of medical advantages kale gives, integrating it into everyday feasts turns into a fundamental undertaking. Reasonable and inventive systems can change kale from a straightforward verdant green into a flexible culinary sidekick that orchestrates wellbeing and flavor. We should investigate viable guidance on flawlessly incorporating kale into the everyday culinary collection, guaranteeing a supported tune of prosperity.

1. **Embrace the Morning Greens: Launch Your Day with a Kale-imbued Breakfast**

   Imbuing the morning schedule with kale establishes an inspirational vibe for the afternoon, giving a supplement pressed establishment that upholds energy and imperativeness. Consider integrating kale into breakfast staples like omelets, scrambles, or breakfast bowls. Sauté hacked kale with onions, tomatoes, and ringer peppers for an energetic and tasty expansion to your morning eggs. On the other hand, mix kale into a morning smoothie, consolidating it with organic products, yogurt, and a hint of honey for a reviving and supplement thick beginning.

   Making a good kale and egg breakfast wrap is another exquisite choice. Sauté kale leaves and crease them into an entire grain tortilla with fried eggs, diced tomatoes, and a sprinkle of cheddar. This basic yet supporting breakfast guarantees that kale becomes the dominant focal point, giving a powerful wholesome profile to launch the day.

2. **Lift Lunch with Kale-implanted Plates of mixed greens and Wraps: A Noontime Supplement Lift**

Noon offers an optimal chance to implant dinners with kale, improving wholesome thickness without compromising flavor. Making kale plates of mixed greens or wraps presents a range of varieties, surfaces, and supplements into the late morning repast.

For a fast and fulfilling kale salad, knead new kale leaves with olive oil, lemon juice, and a spot of salt to mellow the surface. Mix it up of bright vegetables, for example, cherry tomatoes, cucumber cuts, and destroyed carrots. Finish it off with protein sources like barbecued chicken, chickpeas, or quinoa for a balanced and filling feast.

Kale wraps give a helpful and compact lunch choice. Fill an entire grain wrap with a layer of hummus or Greek yogurt, add kale leaves, and incorporate a combination of veggies and lean proteins. Moving it up makes a handheld pleasure that fulfills hunger as well as energizes the body with the healthful extravagance of kale.

3. **Kale as a Culinary Friend in Supper Joys: From Sautéed Greens to Delightful Pastas**

Supper turns into an ideal second to mesh kale into various appetizing and encouraging dishes. Sautéed kale fills in as a fantastic side dish, offering an explosion of flavor and nourishment. In a skillet, heat olive oil, add minced garlic, and throw in cleaved kale leaves. Sauté until shriveled, and wrap up with a press of lemon juice for brilliance. This basic arrangement hoists the dietary substance of any supper plate.

Coordinating kale into pasta dishes acquaints a healthy component with customary recipes. Integrate kale into an entire grain pasta dish by adding it to a sauté of garlic, cherry tomatoes, and white beans. Wrap up with a shower of olive oil and a sprinkle of Parmesan cheddar for a generous and supplement rich supper choice.

Kale can likewise be a star fixing in meals and grain bowls. Layer kale with grains, cooked vegetables, and protein sources like heated chicken or tofu. The outcome is an even and tasty supper that fulfills the sense of taste as well as supports generally wellbeing.

4. **Kale-controlled Nibbling: From Chips to Plunges for Sustaining Breaks**

Nibbling takes on a healthy aspect when kale is integrated into the collection of helpful and fulfilling chomps. Kale chips offer a crunchy and supplement thick option in contrast to conventional bites. Just throw kale leaves with olive oil, sprinkle with ocean salt, and heat until fresh. These custom made kale chips give an irreproachable bite that fulfills desires while adding to day to day supplement consumption.

Matching kale with delightful plunges further improves the nibbling experience.

Kale pesto, made with new kale leaves, garlic, nuts, and Parmesan cheddar, turns into a flexible plunge for entire grain saltines or vegetable sticks. Hummus mixed with kale makes a supplement rich plunge for pita bread or cut cucumbers. These kale-fueled snacks change up day to day snack as well as inject each break with an explosion of wholesome goodness.

5. **Kale in Soups and Stews: Generous and Supplement pressed Solace**
As the weather conditions cools, integrating kale into soups and stews adds a generous and supplement stuffed aspect to soothing feasts. Kale's versatility permits it to hold its surface even in stewing fluids, making it an optimal expansion to different soup recipes.

Kale and white bean soup, for instance, consolidates the verdant green with protein-rich beans, tomatoes, and fragrant spices for a wonderful and sustaining bowl. On the other hand, kale can be highlighted in a vegetable and lentil stew, giving a variety of flavors and surfaces that make every spoonful a healthy enjoyment.

For an extra supplement help, consider adding kale to exemplary chicken noodle soup or minestrone. The dynamic green improves the visual allure as well as contributes an ensemble of nutrients and minerals to the general creation.

6. **Kale-injected Smoothies: A Supplement pressed Taste for Whenever Energy**
Smoothies offer a flexible material for integrating kale into day to day nourishment, giving a helpful and scrumptious method for receiving the rewards of this verdant green. A kale and berry smoothie, for example, mixes kale leaves with a blend of berries, a banana, and a fluid base, for example, almond milk. The outcome is an invigorating and supplement stuffed taste that can be delighted in as a tidbit or a dinner substitution.

For a tropical wind, attempt a kale and pineapple smoothie by joining kale with new pineapple pieces, coconut water, and a bit of ginger. This mix gives an eruption of flavors as well as implants the smoothie with various nutrients and cell reinforcements.

Adding a scoop of protein powder or a dab of Greek yogurt to kale smoothies improves their satiety factor, making them a filling and invigorating choice for breakfast or a post-exercise reward.

7. **Kale as a Pizza Clincher and Wraps: Reexamining Recognizable Top picks**
Reexamining comfortable top choices with kale presents a fun loving and nutritious component to day to day dinners. Rather than customary pizza garnishes, consider adding sautéed kale to pizza for an energetic and supplement pressed curve. Spread a far layer of pureed tomatoes on entire grain hull, add kale leaves, cherry tomatoes, and your #1 cheddar for a delightful and irreproachable pizza choice.

Kale wraps offer an innovative option in contrast to conventional tortillas or flatbreads. Utilize huge kale leaves as a base and fill them with a blend of protein, vegetables, and a tasty sauce. Barbecued chicken or tofu, matched with vivid veggies and a tahini dressing, makes a kale wrap that fulfills the taste buds as well as gives a healthy and adjusted feast.

8. **Frozen Kale for Smoothie Comfort: An Efficient Technique**

   Integrating frozen kale into day to day dinners is an efficient methodology that guarantees comfort without compromising nourishing advantages. Frozen kale is promptly accessible in most supermarkets and can be handily added to smoothies, soups, and stews without the requirement for washing, cleaving, or kneading.

   To make a cooler reserve of frozen kale, wash and completely dry new kale leaves, eliminate the stems, and piece them into cooler cordial sacks or holders. This planning guarantees that frozen kale is promptly accessible for fast and easy fuse into everyday dinners. The flexibility of frozen kale goes with it a pragmatic decision for those looking to smooth out their culinary daily schedule while boosting dietary admission.

9. **Kale-mixed Dressings and Sauces: Delightful Upgrades**

   Hoisting the kind of day to day feasts becomes easy with kale-injected dressings and sauces. Making a basic kale pesto by mixing new kale leaves with garlic, pine nuts, Parmesan cheddar, and olive oil adds an explosion of flavor to pasta dishes, mixed greens, or broiled vegetables. The flexibility of kale pesto stretches out to sandwiches and wraps, making an exquisite and supplement rich fixing.

   Kale-based salad dressings offer one more road for upgrading the flavor profile of new greens. Mix kale with fixings like Greek yogurt, lemon juice, and spices to make a dynamic and tart dressing that hoists the flavor of plates of mixed greens. Sprinkling this kale-mixed dressing over various vegetables and proteins makes an even and tasty feast.

10. **Kale as a Supplement rich Side Dish: A Simple Expansion to Any Plate**

    Making kale a standard side dish is a simple and compelling system for guaranteeing a reliable admission of its nourishing advantages. Sautéed kale with garlic and a sprinkle of olive oil fills in as a speedy and supplement rich side that matches well with different proteins, grains, or pasta dishes. The effortlessness of this readiness permits kale to supplement a large number of fundamental courses without eclipsing their flavors.

    For a bend on conventional side dishes, consider kale gratin — a heated goulash highlighting kale, cheddar, and breadcrumbs. This tasty and consoling dish not just adds a nourishing lift to the plate yet in addition presents a new and creative method for getting a charge out of kale as a component of the day to day feasting experience.

11. **Kale as a Trimming: Adding Nourishing Pizazz to Each Dish**

    Raising the visual allure of feasts while adding a nourishing pizazz becomes easy with kale as an embellishment. Utilize finely slashed kale as a beautiful and supplement rich garnish for soups, stews, and mixed greens. The dynamic green tint of kale upgrades the introduction of dishes, making them outwardly engaging and welcoming.

Sprinkle hacked kale over breakfast bowls, yogurt parfaits, or even appetizing dishes like heated yams. This straightforward expansion contributes an explosion of newness as well as presents the wholesome orchestra of kale to each chomp. The flexibility of kale as a trimming considers innovative trial and error, giving a chance to implant each dinner with both stylish and healthy benefit.

12. Developing Your Own Kale: An Economical Methodology

For those with the means and tendency, developing kale at home offers a manageable way to deal with integrating this verdant green into day to day feasts. Kale is a tough and strong plant that flourishes in different environments, making it reasonable for home nurseries. Establishing kale seeds or seedlings in a nursery bed or holders gives a ceaseless stockpile of new kale leaves.

Local kale not just guarantees a prepared and helpful wellspring of this nutritious green yet additionally encourages a more profound association with the food we eat. Reaping kale from one's own nursery adds a feeling of satisfaction and manageability to the day to day culinary experience, building up the possibility that healthy nourishment can be developed and delighted in inside the solace of one's home.

Developing a Supported Song of Prosperity with Kale

Integrating kale into everyday feasts is an excursion of culinary investigation and dietary insight. The down to earth exhortation offered envelops a range of innovative and open methodologies, guaranteeing that kale turns into a consistent and charming piece of the day to day eating experience. From morning greens to generous meals, kale-imbued snacks to supplement stuffed smoothies, the flexibility of kale permits it to orchestrate with different foods and culinary inclinations.

As people embrace the down to earth ways to integrate kale into everyday feasts, they effectively partake in developing a supported song of prosperity. The supplement rich orchestra of nutrients, minerals, and phytonutrients inside kale adds to by and large wellbeing and imperativeness. Whether delighted in a lively serving of mixed greens, mixed into a reviving smoothie, or sautéed as an exquisite side, kale turns out to be in excess of a verdant green — it changes into a culinary buddy that reverberates with the standards of comprehensive prosperity.

In the kale-mixed day to day daily schedule, people support their bodies as well as praise the delight of healthy eating. Every feast turns into a valuable chance to relish the flavors, colors, and wholesome advantages of kale — a verdant green that adds both liveliness and sustenance to the orchestra of day to day living. In developing a supported song of prosperity with kale, people set out on a culinary excursion that reaches out past sustenance — it turns into a festival of wellbeing, imagination, and the persevering through delight of enjoying an everyday routine very much experienced.

4.3 Real-life success stories of individuals experiencing lung health improvements

Breathing Recharged: Genuine Accounts of Lung Wellbeing Wins

In the embroidered artwork of human encounters, accounts of win over lung wellbeing provokes stand as strong tributes to the strength of the human soul. Genuine examples of overcoming adversity enlighten the excursion of people who, against chances and impediments, have explored the way to further developed lung wellbeing. These stories reverberate with trust, constancy, and the groundbreaking effect of way of life changes, clinical intercessions, and the faithful soul of the individuals who have set out on the excursion to inhale recharged. Allow us to dive into the motivating narratives of people whose lives have been moved by the quest for lung wellbeing upgrades.

Story 1: From Windedness to Breathing Effortlessness

John, a 55-year-old eager climber, found his enthusiasm for the paths suddenly ended by industrious windedness. Concerned, he looked for clinical exhortation and was determined to have constant obstructive pneumonic illness (COPD), a condition described by impeded wind current to the lungs. Not entirely settled, John teamed up with his medical services group to foster a far reaching technique for lung wellbeing improvement.

Under the direction of his pulmonologist, John embraced a multi-layered approach. Respiratory restoration turned into a foundation of his excursion, integrating breathing activities, high-impact molding, and strength preparing into his daily schedule. With the backing of a respiratory specialist, he learned methods to upgrade his breathing examples and oversee side effects.

Notwithstanding organized work out, John made way of life changes, focusing on a supplement rich eating routine to help generally prosperity. Expanded utilization of natural products, vegetables, and lean proteins became essential to his day to day decisions. Besides, he quit smoking, a urgent move toward easing back the movement of COPD.

Over the long run, John's responsibility proved to be fruitful. He saw a continuous improvement in his capacity to inhale, set apart by expanded endurance and diminished episodes of shortness of breath. Normal observing with his medical care group considered acclimations to his therapy plan, guaranteeing that he kept on advancing on the way to lung wellbeing. Yet again today, John partakes in the paths as well as fills in as a backer for respiratory wellbeing, sharing his excursion to motivate others confronting comparative difficulties.

Story 2: An Excursion from Asthma Limitations to Dynamic Living

Sarah, a dynamic 30-year-old, had gone through a lot of her time on earth exploring the imperatives of asthma. Continuous episodes of wheezing and windedness restricted her cooperation in proactive tasks and outside pursuits. Still up in the air to break liberated from the limitations forced by her condition, Sarah set out on a proactive excursion toward better lung wellbeing.

Instructing herself about asthma triggers and the executives methodologies turned into an essential initial step. Outfitted with information, she teamed up intimately with her allergist to recognize explicit triggers and foster a customized activity plan. Sarah's obligation to following her recommended meds reliably assumed a critical part in dealing with her side effects successfully.

Perceiving the cooperative connection between actual work and respiratory wellbeing, Sarah step by step integrated practice into her daily schedule. Beginning with low-influence exercises, for example, strolling and yoga, she continuously expanded the power and term of her exercises. Quite, she viewed swimming as especially helpful, as the moist climate demonstrated relieving to her aviation routes.

Notwithstanding pharmacological mediations and exercise, Sarah focused on ecological changes. Carrying out measures to decrease allergens in her living space, like utilizing air purifiers and limiting openness to triggers, added to a huge decrease in asthma intensifications.

Sarah's obligation to her lung wellbeing changed her day to day existence as well as opened ways to additional opportunities. She turned into a backer for asthma mindfulness, sharing her encounters to engage others confronting comparative difficulties. Today, Sarah drives a functioning way of life, partaking in long distance races and open air experiences, and fills in as a motivation to those exploring the excursion toward further developed lung wellbeing.

Story 3: Beating Aspiratory Difficulties through Pneumonic Recovery

Mark, a 65-year-old retired person, confronted the overwhelming test of remaking his life after an ongoing lung condition left him incapacitated. Determined to have interstitial lung infection, an ever-evolving condition influencing the lung tissue, Imprint's day to day exercises were seriously confined by steady shortness of breath and exhaustion. Baffled by the limits forced by his condition, he went to pneumonic restoration as an encouraging sign.

Under the direction of a multidisciplinary group, including pulmonologists, respiratory specialists, and exercise physiologists, Imprint left on an organized pneumonic restoration program. The program zeroed in on upgrading his actual perseverance, improving his breathing mechanics, and offering profound help through guiding and schooling.

The activity part of pneumonic restoration turned into an extraordinary component in Imprint's excursion. Managed oxygen consuming activities, strength preparing, and breathing activities were custom fitted to his particular necessities and continuously advanced as his lung capability permitted. Standard checking and acclimations to the activity routine guaranteed a protected and powerful way to deal with recovery.

Past the actual angles, Imprint found comfort in the mental help presented by the pneumonic recovery program. Directing meetings gave a space to address the inner difficulties related with persistent lung conditions, encouraging flexibility and a positive mentality.

Imprint's devotion to aspiratory recovery yielded noteworthy outcomes. Over the long run, he encountered expanded endurance, a decrease in shortness of breath, and an upgraded capacity to perform exercises of everyday living. His excursion featured the advantages of organized restoration as well as highlighted the significance of a far reaching approach that tends to both physical and close to home parts of lung wellbeing.

Story 4: A Groundbreaking Excursion through Comprehensive Way of life Changes

Emma, a 40-year-old mother of two, confronted an overwhelming conclusion of idiopathic pneumonic fibrosis (IPF), an ever-evolving lung illness with no known fix.

Not entirely settled to upgrade her personal satisfaction, Emma embraced an all encompassing way to deal with lung wellbeing, incorporating way of life changes that stretched out past clinical mediations.

Fundamental to Emma's methodology was a pledge to healthful greatness. She teamed up with an enlisted dietitian to make an eating regimen wealthy in calming food sources, cell reinforcements, and fundamental supplements. Underscoring a plant-based diet with various organic products, vegetables, and entire grains turned into a foundation of her everyday decisions. Emma's eating routine likewise included food sources with potential lung medical advantages, for example, omega-3 unsaturated fats tracked down in greasy fish.

Actual work assumed a fundamental part in Emma's excursion. Regardless of the difficulties presented by her condition, she took part in delicate activities, including strolling, yoga, and kendo. The attention was on advancing adaptability, keeping up with muscle strength, and enhancing by and large prosperity.

Mind-body works on, including reflection and stress the board, became necessary parts of Emma's everyday daily schedule. Perceiving the interconnectedness of mental and actual wellbeing, she focused on exercises that encouraged unwinding and profound prosperity.

Emma's process likewise elaborate dynamic cooperation in help gatherings and promotion endeavors inside the pneumonic fibrosis local area. Interfacing with others confronting comparable difficulties gave a feeling of brotherhood and common help, supporting the significance of a local area in the excursion toward further developed lung wellbeing.

While Emma's condition stays an everyday test, her obligation to a comprehensive methodology has yielded substantial advantages. She encounters a greater of life, decreased feelings of anxiety, and a feeling of strengthening in effectively dealing with her wellbeing. Emma's story highlights the groundbreaking capability of way of life changes despite constant lung conditions, filling in as a motivation to those looking for far reaching techniques for lung wellbeing improvement.

Story 5: An Excursion from Inactive Way of life to Respiratory Versatility

Meet Alex, a 45-year-seasoned pro with a background marked by an inactive way of life and incidental smoking. Unbeknownst to him, his lung wellbeing was progressively compromised throughout the long term, prompting a finding of beginning phase persistent bronchitis. Confronted with the obvious truth of his respiratory wellbeing, Alex chose to revamp his account by focusing on actual work and way of life changes.

At first reluctant and overwhelmed by the possibility of taking on a more dynamic way of life, Alex took little, purposeful advances. He started with short strolls around his area, slowly expanding both distance and speed as his perseverance moved along. Taking part in outside exercises, like cycling and climbing, became wellsprings of happiness and inspiration.

Urgently, Alex looked for direction from a wellness coach experienced in working with people with respiratory circumstances. Together, they fostered a customized practice plan that consolidated cardiovascular exercises, strength preparing, and breathing activities. The organized methodology upgraded Alex's actual wellness as well as imparted trust in his capacity to oversee and work on his respiratory wellbeing.

Couple with active work, Alex upgraded his eating routine, consolidating food sources known for their lung-accommodating properties. New products of the soil, especially those wealthy in cancer prevention agents, became staples of his dinners. He decreased handled food sources and embraced a more adjusted and supplement thick eating routine, perceiving the harmonious connection among sustenance and respiratory prosperity.

As the months passed, Alex saw huge upgrades in his lung capability and generally prosperity. Windedness turned out to be less incessant, and he encountered expanded energy levels that gushed out over into different parts of his life. Alex's process epitomizes the groundbreaking effect of embracing a functioning way of life and pursuing cognizant dietary decisions in advancing lung wellbeing.

Story 6: Reversing the situation of Respiratory Difficulties with All encompassing Treatments

Rachel, a 50-year-old yoga teacher, ended up wrestling with steady respiratory issues, at last analyzed as asthma exacerbated by pressure. Still up in the air to find a comprehensive arrangement, Rachel set out on an excursion that flawlessly coordinated her mastery in yoga with conventional clinical mediations.

Perceiving the significance of stress the board in relieving her asthma side effects, Rachel focused on yoga and contemplation in her day to day everyday practice. Breathing activities, known as pranayama, turned into a foundation of her training. These deliberate breathwork meetings quieted her sensory system as well as worked on her respiratory limit over the long haul.

Rachel worked together with her medical services group to make a far reaching asthma the board plan that included both pharmacological intercessions and all encompassing methodologies. Under the oversight of her pulmonologist, she step by step diminished dependence on salvage inhalers and found that her asthma assaults turned out to be less incessant and less extreme.

Notwithstanding her own excursion, Rachel started integrating respiratory-centered yoga classes into her educating collection. These specific classes took care of people with respiratory circumstances, offering a strong climate for them to investigate the advantages of careful development and breath mindfulness.

Rachel's obligation to an all encompassing methodology stretched out past her own and proficient life. She turned into a supporter for the reconciliation of corresponding treatments in respiratory consideration, underscoring the significance of customized, patient-focused approaches. Her story embodies the expected collaboration between traditional medication and all encompassing practices in accomplishing respiratory versatility.

Story 7: Exploring Pediatric Respiratory Difficulties with Family Backing

The excursion toward further developed lung wellbeing isn't selective to grown-ups. Sarah, a mother of a six-year-old kid named Noah, wound up confronting the difficulties of dealing with Noah's asthma determination. Still up in the air to furnish her child with the most ideal consideration, Sarah embraced a family-focused way to deal with help Noah's respiratory prosperity.

Training assumed an essential part in Sarah's procedure. She worked intimately with Noah's pediatrician to grasp the triggers and the board strategies intended for pediatric asthma. Furnished with information, she engaged Noah to turn into a functioning member in his own consideration, showing him the significance of taking recommended drugs and perceiving early indications of asthma compounding.

As a family, they carried out natural changes to make an asthma-accommodating home. Sarah guaranteed normal cleaning to limit allergens, and they assigned explicit regions as without smoke zones. Furthermore, they developed a steady climate where Noah felt happy with communicating his interests about his respiratory wellbeing.

Actual work turned into an essential piece of Noah's daily practice, with the family taking part in outside exercises that advanced both activity and delight. Sarah looked for direction from Noah's medical services group to distinguish appropriate proactive tasks that lined up with his respiratory necessities. This family-situated approach upheld Noah's lung wellbeing as well as cultivated a feeling of solidarity and versatility inside the family.

Sarah's support stretched out to Noah's school climate, where she teamed up with instructors to make an asthma-accommodating arrangement. Educators and staff were instructed about Noah's condition, and an arrangement was laid out to address potential asthma triggers during school hours. Sarah's proactive methodology guaranteed that Noah could flourish scholastically while dealing with his respiratory wellbeing actually.

Noah's process fills in as an update that pediatric respiratory difficulties require an all encompassing and family-focused approach. Through training, backing, and support, families can explore the intricacies of pediatric asthma, permitting kids like Noah to lead dynamic and satisfying lives.

An Ensemble of Versatility in Lung Wellbeing Excursions

In the continuation of genuine examples of overcoming adversity, the stories of Alex, Rachel, and Sarah and Noah reverberation the orchestra of flexibility that penetrates lung wellbeing ventures. Every story represents the special ways people and families navigate in their quest for worked on respiratory prosperity.

These extra stories spotlight the groundbreaking capability of way of life changes, all encompassing treatments, and family-focused approaches in the domain of lung wellbeing. They highlight the variety of procedures people utilize, underlining that there is nobody size-fits-all answer for respiratory difficulties.

As the orchestra of flexibility in lung wellbeing ventures keeps on unfurling, these accounts add to an aggregate story of trust, strengthening, and the persevering through soul of the people who decide to focus on their respiratory prosperity. Whether through actual work, all encompassing practices, or family support, these accounts represent the multi-layered approaches that can prompt breathing recharged.

Chapter 5

Turmeric Interlude Anti-inflammatory Support for Lungs

Turmeric Interval: Mitigating Backing for Lungs

In the complex embroidery of wellbeing and prosperity, the energetic tones of turmeric arise as a strong break, offering an orchestra of mitigating support for the lungs. Past its culinary charm, turmeric, a brilliant tinted zest got from the Curcuma longa plant, harbors a gold mine of bioactive mixtures, with curcumin becoming the overwhelming focus. This recess dives into the multi-layered job of turmeric in offering mitigating help for respiratory wellbeing, investigating its verifiable roots, logical underpinnings, and functional applications in advancing lung prosperity.

Authentic Roots: Turmeric's Process through Time

The excursion of turmeric follows back hundreds of years, woven into the social and restorative embroidered artwork of old civilizations.

Beginning from Southeast Asia, turmeric tracked down its direction into Ayurveda, the customary medication arrangement of India, where it was respected for its multi-layered restorative properties. Turmeric turned into a staple in Ayurvedic definitions, praised for its calming, cell reinforcement, and resistant tweaking credits.

The authentic meaning of turmeric rises above the Indian subcontinent, arriving at all over across assorted societies. In customary Chinese medication, turmeric was embraced for its job in strengthening course and tending to conditions related with irritation. The flavor likewise cut its place in customary recuperating rehearses in locales going from the Center East to Africa, each culture mixing turmeric with its extraordinary restorative setting.

As hundreds of years unfurled, turmeric crossed mainlands, finding its direction into culinary practices and natural pharmacists the same. The brilliant powder turned into a culinary chemist's device, implanting dishes with both flavor and wellbeing advancing properties. Today, the verifiable tradition of turmeric perseveres as a demonstration of its getting through importance in the domain of all encompassing prosperity.

Logical Underpinnings: Divulging the Force of Curcumin

At the core of turmeric's restorative ability lies curcumin, a polyphenolic compound that fills in as its essential bioactive constituent. Curcumin, with its powerful mitigating and cancer prevention agent credits, has turned into the subject of broad logical investigation, spellbinding analysts and wellbeing devotees the same.

The calming systems of curcumin are diverse, affecting different atomic pathways associated with the provocative reaction. It balances the movement of key compounds and flagging particles, downregulating incendiary arbiters and checking the fountain of favorable to provocative occasions. Moreover, curcumin shows cell reinforcement properties, killing free revolutionaries and oxidative pressure that can add to irritation.

Logical examinations have divulged curcumin's true capacity in alleviating constant fiery circumstances, including those influencing the respiratory framework. Conditions like persistent obstructive pneumonic illness (COPD), asthma, and interstitial lung infection include provocative cycles, and curcumin's modulatory consequences for irritation offer a promising road for helpful investigation.

Notwithstanding its calming ability, curcumin shows immunomodulatory impacts, impacting the movement of invulnerable cells and adding to a reasonable insusceptible reaction. This double limit — fighting irritation while supporting safe capability — positions curcumin as a flexible partner in the multifaceted dance of keeping up with respiratory wellbeing.

Commonsense Applications: Turmeric's Respiratory Reverberation

As the logical comprehension of turmeric's advantages extends, viable applications for respiratory prosperity come to the front. Integrating turmeric into day to day schedules can take different structures, each offering a delectable and restorative intermission for the lungs.

Brilliant Elixirs of Wellbeing: Turmeric Tea and Lattes

Turmeric tea, frequently alluded to as brilliant tea, fills in as a calming solution that consolidates the glow of flavors with the mitigating properties of turmeric. The planning includes stewing turmeric, ginger, cinnamon, and different flavors in water, making a fragrant mixture. This brilliant remedy pleases the faculties as well as gives a soothing and calming stop for the respiratory framework.

Turmeric lattes, or brilliant lattes, present a cutting edge wind, mixing turmeric with milk (dairy or plant-based), a bit of sugar, and sweet-smelling flavors. The outcome is a rich and sustaining drink that can be delighted in as a quieting custom, offering respiratory help with each taste.

Curcumin-Rich Culinary Manifestations: From Brilliant Curries to Turmeric-mixed Dishes

In the domain of culinary imagination, turmeric becomes the dominant focal point in a range of dishes. Brilliant curries, where turmeric mixes its brilliant tint into rich and delightful stews, grandstand the flavor's adaptability. Integrating turmeric into vegetable sautés, rice dishes, and soups confers lively variety as well as presents a gustatory orchestra that reverberates with stimulating advantages.

Turmeric's bioavailability can be improved by matching it with dark pepper, which contains piperine — a compound known to work with the ingestion of curcumin. This unique team, frequently found in customary curry mixes, makes a cooperative energy that expands the bioactive capability of turmeric.

Turmeric Enhancements: Containers and Concentrates for Designated Help

Perceiving the viable difficulties of integrating turmeric into each dinner, numerous people go to turmeric supplements for designated respiratory help. Turmeric cases, containing normalized curcumin separates, offer a helpful and concentrated type of the flavor's remedial mixtures.

While picking turmeric supplements, factors like bioavailability, nature of extraction, and the presence of extra fixings ought to be thought of. A few plans incorporate dark pepper concentrate to upgrade curcumin ingestion, guaranteeing that the enhancement really conveys its mitigating benefits.

Do-It-Yourself Turmeric Covers: Supporting Respiratory Health Through the Skin

Past the domain of culinary enjoyments, turmeric stretches out its impact to skincare ceremonies. Do-It-Yourself turmeric covers, joining turmeric with fixings like yogurt, honey, and aloe vera, offer a comprehensive way to deal with respiratory well-being through the skin.

Applied as a facial covering, turmeric's calming and cell reinforcement properties can mitigate and support the skin, adding to a feeling of generally speaking prosperity.

While the essential focal point of such covers is skincare, the demonstration of taking care of oneself and the retention of turmeric's bioactive mixtures through the skin add a nuanced layer to the respiratory break. As the skin ingests the gainful properties of turmeric, the tactile experience turns into a delicate indication of the interconnectedness between outer ceremonies and interior prosperity.

Exploring Contemplations: Turmeric's Concordance with Wellbeing

While turmeric remains as a flexible partner in the journey for respiratory prosperity, certain contemplations ought to be recognized. Individual reactions to turmeric can change, and it is prudent to talk with medical services experts, particularly for those with existing ailments or those taking meds. Turmeric, in culinary amounts, is by and large viewed as safe for most people, however high portions from enhancements might connect with specific drugs or have contraindications.

Moreover, the bioavailability of curcumin, the dynamic compound in turmeric, can be restricted. Consolidating turmeric with dark pepper, as generally finished in curry mixes, can improve retention. Moreover, the presence of fats in a feast can additionally work with curcumin retention, making turmeric a brilliant option to dishes cooked with oils or fats.

Pregnant people and those with gallbladder issues ought to practice mindfulness and look for customized exhortation in regards to turmeric utilization. While turmeric is praised for its bunch benefits, an individualized and adjusted approach guarantees its amicable mix into one's wellbeing process.

Turmeric's Radiant Notes in the Respiratory Orchestra

As we explore the complicated orchestra of respiratory prosperity, the dazzling notes of turmeric arise as an agreeable recess, offering calming support and an embroidery of energizing advantages. From its verifiable roots saturated with conventional medication to its cutting edge applications in culinary manifestations and enhancements, turmeric remains as a flexible partner chasing lung wellbeing.

The logical underpinnings of turmeric, with curcumin at the front, enlighten its ability to adjust aggravation and backing invulnerable capability. Useful applications, going from brilliant elixirs and culinary enjoyments to skincare ceremonies, give people assorted roads to integrate turmeric into their regular routines.

Similarly as with any wellbeing venture, an individualized and adjusted approach guarantees that turmeric's brilliant notes fit with's one of a kind wellbeing needs. As the centuries progressed, turmeric has navigated social scenes, making a permanent imprint on the all encompassing quest for prosperity. Today, its brilliant presence in the respiratory orchestra welcomes people to embrace the glow, flavor, and restorative reverberation of this immortal zest, meshing turmeric's radiant strings into the texture of lung wellbeing.

5.1 Uncover the anti-inflammatory benefits of turmeric

Revealing the Mitigating Embroidery of Turmeric: An Orchestra of Health

In the domain of comprehensive wellbeing, scarcely any normal substances enamor the creative mind and logical interest as much as turmeric. This brilliant shaded zest, got from the Curcuma longa plant, has been loved for quite a long time, for its culinary lavishness as well as for its powerful restorative properties. At the core of turmeric's remedial charm lies curcumin, a bioactive compound that winds around a many-sided embroidery of mitigating benefits. This investigation dives into the diverse idea of turmeric's calming ability, unwinding its verifiable roots, logical underpinnings, and functional applications in cultivating in general prosperity.

Authentic Adoration: Turmeric's Process Through Time

Turmeric's process through time is saturated with the rich customs of old human advancements, especially in the Indian subcontinent. As a foundation of Ayurveda, the conventional medication arrangement of India, turmeric became inseparable from health and essentialness. Its utilization goes back north of 4,000 years, where it was embraced as a culinary flavor as well as a remedial specialist for a heap of sicknesses.

The authentic respect for turmeric rises above borders, finding reverberations in conventional recuperating rehearses across different societies. In customary Chinese medication, turmeric was esteemed for its capacity to animate dissemination and ease conditions related with irritation. The flavor's brilliant gleam embellished Center

Eastern mending customs, and it ventured across mainlands, making a permanent imprint on culinary and restorative scenes.

Since forever ago, turmeric has been in excess of a simple flavor; it has been an image of wellbeing, a healer in different definitions, and a demonstration of the old insight that perceived the harmonious connection among nature and prosperity. The verifiable underlying foundations of turmeric establish the groundwork for its proceeded with importance in contemporary comprehensive wellbeing rehearses.

Logical Light: Deciphering the Force of Curcumin

In the lab, the spotlight goes to curcumin, the essential bioactive compound inside turmeric answerable for its exceptional medical advantages. The logical investigation of curcumin's properties has uncovered an abundance of information in regards to its mitigating components and expected remedial applications.

At the sub-atomic level, curcumin applies its mitigating impacts by tweaking different flagging pathways and sub-atomic targets. It hinders the movement of key compounds associated with the provocative interaction, checking the creation of incendiary go betweens. Furthermore, curcumin shows cancer prevention agent properties, killing free revolutionaries that add to irritation and oxidative pressure.

Various examinations have dove into curcumin's true capacity in tending to persistent fiery circumstances, going from joint pain to cardiovascular illnesses. With regards to respiratory wellbeing, where irritation assumes a crucial part in conditions like asthma, constant obstructive pneumonic sickness (COPD), and interstitial lung illness, curcumin arises as a promising contender for restorative mediation.

The safe regulating impacts of curcumin further add to its mitigating profile. By impacting the action of resistant cells, curcumin keeps a reasonable invulnerable reaction. This double limit — restraining irritation while supporting resistant capability — renders curcumin a flexible partner in the mission for in general wellbeing.

Commonsense Application: Turmeric's Adaptability in Regular Wellbeing

The commonsense utilization of turmeric's calming benefits stretches out across different features of day to day existence, offering an orchestra of choices that take special care of individual inclinations and ways of life.

Culinary Enjoyments: From Brilliant Lattes to Turmeric-implanted Cooking

In kitchens all over the planet, turmeric becomes the dominant focal point, implanting dishes with its warm, gritty flavor and dynamic tone. Brilliant lattes, mixing turmeric with milk and sweet-smelling flavors, offer a consoling and calming refreshment. This cutting edge variation of customary turmeric tea has turned into a wellbeing custom, wedding flavor with stimulating guilty pleasure.

Turmeric's culinary flexibility reaches out past drinks. From brilliant curries that elegance supper tables to turmeric-injected soups, stews, and even sweets, the zest fits a variety of culinary manifestations. The consideration of dark pepper in curry mixes improves the bioavailability of curcumin, guaranteeing that its calming benefits are amplified.

Supplemental Help: Outfitting Curcumin's Concentrated Power

Perceiving the useful difficulties of integrating turmeric into each feast, numerous people go to turmeric supplements for designated help. Cases containing normalized curcumin removes give a concentrated type of the flavor's remedial mixtures. These enhancements, when taken in suitable portions, offer a helpful road for people trying to outfit the mitigating advantages of curcumin.

It's fundamental to think about variables like the nature of extraction, bioavailability, and expected collaborations with drugs while choosing turmeric supplements. A few details incorporate piperine, the dynamic compound in dark pepper, to improve curcumin retention.

Effective Treats: Turmeric Covers for Skin and Then some

Turmeric's excursion from the kitchen to the restroom includes skincare ceremonies that stretch out past the surface. Do-It-Yourself turmeric covers, made with fixings like yogurt, honey, and aloe vera, offer a tactile encounter that goes past shallow. While these covers essentially address skincare concerns, the ingestion of curcumin through the skin adds a nuanced layer to the calming intermission.

Turmeric's calming and cell reinforcement properties add to a relieving and supporting impact on the skin. As people enjoy these skincare customs, they participate in an exemplification of all encompassing prosperity, where the outer and interior domains unite in an amicable dance.

Culinary Speculative chemistry: Improving Bioavailability with Synergistic Fixings

Turmeric's bioavailability, the degree to which the body can assimilate and use its dynamic mixtures, can be affected by the culinary speculative chemistry of matching it with specific fixings. The consideration of fats, for example, those tracked down in oils or ghee, upgrades the assimilation of curcumin. Besides, consolidating turmeric with dark pepper, which contains piperine, makes a synergistic impact that further lifts bioavailability.

Investigating culinary practices that embrace these collaborations —, for example, the matching of turmeric with coconut milk in customary Indian food — gives a brilliant tangible encounter as well as an essential way to deal with enhancing the mitigating advantages of turmeric.

Exploring Contemplations: Turmeric's Amicable Incorporation

While turmeric offers a plenty of medical advantages, its amicable incorporation into health rehearses requires smart thought. Individual reactions to turmeric can change, and certain contemplations ought to be remembered, particularly for those with previous ailments or those taking prescriptions.

Turmeric, in its culinary structure, is by and large safe for most people when consumed in moderate amounts. In any case, high dosages from enhancements might associate with specific meds or have contraindications. Talking with medical care experts guarantees customized guidance that lines up with individual wellbeing needs.

Moreover, pregnant people and those with gallbladder issues ought to practice mindfulness and look for direction in regards to turmeric utilization. While turmeric is praised for its bunch benefits, an individualized and adjusted approach guarantees its agreeable incorporation into one's wellbeing process.

Turmeric's Immortal Reverberation in Health

In the ensemble of comprehensive health, turmeric's immortal reverberation reverberations through the passageways of history, science, and ordinary living. The mitigating advantages of turmeric, coordinated by the virtuosity of curcumin, have situated this brilliant zest as a robust sidekick chasing prosperity.

The verifiable love for turmeric, profoundly imbued in social practices, entwines with the logical light that disentangles the sub-atomic complexities of curcumin. From the kitchens where brilliant lattes are made to the enhancement cases that exemplify curcumin's concentrated power, turmeric's adaptability permits people to fit its mitigating advantages to their exceptional inclinations and ways of life.

As turmeric's brilliant tints decorate culinary manifestations, skincare customs, and supplemental regimens, its amicable combination into wellbeing rehearses requires a careful methodology. Exploring contemplations and looking for customized exhortation guarantees that the ensemble of turmeric's advantages adjusts flawlessly with individual wellbeing needs.

In the excellent embroidery of comprehensive wellbeing, turmeric remains as a signal of versatility — a brilliant string that winds through time, societies, and the different scenes of prosperity. Its immortal reverberation welcomes people to participate in the orchestra of health, where the mitigating notes of turmeric play an agreeable tune — a tune that rises above the limits of custom and science, resounding with the pith of all encompassing residing.

5.2 Culinary techniques to include turmeric in diverse dishes

Culinary Masterfulness with Turmeric: Lifting Dishes with Brilliant Brilliance

In the domain of culinary investigation, turmeric arises as a brilliant star, conferring not exclusively its brilliant tint yet additionally an embroidery of flavors and stimulating advantages to a bunch of dishes. The culinary strategies utilized to integrate turmeric into different foods and recipes lift the specialty of cooking, transforming it into an energetic and wellbeing cognizant undertaking. This investigation dives into the flexible universe of culinary procedures that embrace turmeric, offering an orchestra of potential outcomes to imbue dishes with both variety and health.

1. **Injecting Brilliant Elixirs: Turmeric Teas and Lattes**

   Turmeric's excursion in the kitchen frequently starts with the production of brilliant elixirs that enamor both the faculties and the soul. Turmeric teas and lattes are significant of this sly imbuement, giving an encouraging and refreshing custom.

   To create a turmeric tea, one can begin by stewing water with turmeric, ginger, and other fragrant flavors. This mixture brings about a fragrant remedy that can be delighted in all alone or with a bit of honey for pleasantness.

Turmeric lattes, a cutting edge variation, include mixing turmeric with milk (dairy or plant-based), a touch of sugar, and flavors like cinnamon or cardamom. The outcome is a smooth, brilliant drink that charms the taste buds as well as offers calming benefits.

2. **Brilliant Curries: A Culinary Material**

   Turmeric's job in curries is notable, and the craft of making brilliant toned works of art reaches out across different culinary practices. Whether it's an exemplary Indian curry, a Thai coconut curry, or a Center Eastern stew, turmeric fills in as a foundation in creating an energetic and delightful base.

   The strategy includes sautéing turmeric in oil or ghee toward the start of the cooking system. This not just bestows its brilliant variety to the dish yet in addition permits the fat-solvent mixtures in turmeric, including curcumin, to imbue the whole creation. The expansion of different flavors, spices, and fixings further forms layers of intricacy, making a culinary material that grandstands both creativity and wellbeing.

3. **Turmeric-Implanted Rice and Grains: Enjoying Brilliance**

   Rice and grains, central staples in numerous foods, become a material for turmeric's brilliant brilliance. Turmeric-injected rice adds visual enticement for a dish as well as confers an inconspicuous natural flavor.

   The method includes sautéing crude rice in turmeric-implanted oil prior to cooking. This straightforward yet compelling step changes the whole person of the rice, making a lively side dish that matches perfectly with a scope of principal courses. Likewise, integrating turmeric into quinoa, couscous, or different grains upgrades their variety as well as their wholesome profile, adding a dash of health to each nibble.

4. **Turmeric Zest Mixes: Making Delightful Speculative chemistry**

   Making customized zest mixes that include turmeric permits culinary fans to inject different dishes with an eruption of flavor. Customary zest mixes like curry powder frequently incorporate turmeric, alongside other integral flavors like cumin, coriander, and fenugreek.

   The procedure includes toasting entire flavors and crushing them along with turmeric to make a fragrant and delightful powder. This flavor mix can then be integrated into different recipes, from soups and stews to marinades and rubs for meats or vegetables. The flexibility of turmeric in zest mixes enables cooks to explore different avenues regarding flavor profiles that line up with their culinary inclinations.

5. **Turmeric Sauces and Dressings: Delectable Brilliant Showers**

   Sauces and dressings give a material to turmeric to communicate its culinary flexibility, lifting the flavor profile of a dish with a delicious brilliant shower.

From tart turmeric vinaigrettes to smooth turmeric tahini sauces, the choices are different and magnificent.

Making a turmeric-based sauce frequently includes mixing the flavor with fixings like olive oil, lemon juice, garlic, and spices. The subsequent sauce can be utilized as a marinade for proteins, a sprinkle for cooked vegetables, or a dressing for servings of mixed greens. This method not just improves the visual allure of the dish yet additionally presents an eruption of flavor and invigorating mixtures.

6. **Turmeric in Baking: Brilliant Twists**

The universe of baking greets turmeric wholeheartedly, welcoming its brilliant brilliance to upgrade both the visual allure and dietary benefit of prepared merchandise. From brilliant shaded bread and moves to turmeric-implanted treats and cakes, this culinary method offers an inventive wind to customary recipes.

Integrating turmeric into heated merchandise frequently includes adding the zest to the dry fixings, guaranteeing an even appropriation all through the player. This procedure permits the warm and gritty notes of turmeric to supplement the pleasantness of prepared treats, making an agreeable combination of flavors. Furthermore, the calming advantages of turmeric add a wellbeing component to liberal pleasures.

7. **Turmeric Pickling: Protecting Dynamic quality**

Protecting the dynamic quality of turmeric stretches out past its culinary use in pickling. Turmeric pickles, with their splendid variety and intense flavor, act as a fiery sauce that supplements a scope of dishes.

The strategy includes consolidating turmeric with other pickling fixings like vinegar, salt, and flavors. The outcome is a tart and interesting pickle that can be delighted in close by exquisite dishes or utilized as a tasty expansion to sandwiches and mixed greens. This pickling strategy protects turmeric's brilliant brilliance as well as presents an eruption of sharpness and intricacy to the sense of taste.

8. **Turmeric Treats: Sweet Brilliant Guilty pleasure**

The universe of treats turns into a domain of sweet brilliant guilty pleasure with the consideration of turmeric. From turmeric-flavored frozen yogurts to brilliant milk panna cottas, the zest loans its glow and heartiness to different sweet manifestations.

Integrating turmeric into sweets frequently includes implanting it into creams, custards, or syrups. This method permits the sweet notes of pastries to orchestrate with the unpretentious fieriness of turmeric, making an even and captivating flavor profile. The brilliant shade of turmeric adds visual charm to pastries, transforming every sweet chomp into a tactile encounter.

9. **Turmeric in Aging: Probiotic Brilliance**

The maturation interaction invites turmeric as a lively expansion to pickles, krauts, and other aged delights. Turmeric's gritty flavor coordinates well with the tartness of matured food varieties, making a collaboration that adds profundity and intricacy.

The method includes adding turmeric to vegetables during the maturation cycle, permitting its flavor to implant the whole group. This not just gives a brilliant tint to the matured products yet additionally presents the potential medical advantages related with both turmeric and the probiotics created during maturation. The outcome is a delightful and stimulating expansion to the universe of matured food varieties.

10. **Turmeric-Injected Drinks: Extinguishing Wellbeing**

Drinks, both hot and cool, become a material for turmeric's brilliant mixture, offering an invigorating and restorative method for remaining hydrated. From turmeric-imbued lemonades to chilled turmeric teas, these drinks furnish an extinguishing break with a smidgen of wellbeing.

The procedure includes integrating turmeric into refreshment recipes, whether through mixtures, syrups, or mixed creations. Turmeric's warm and somewhat unpleasant notes supplement the pleasantness of products of the soil freshness of spices, making a different scope of drinks that take care of different taste inclinations. Moreover, the mitigating properties of turmeric add an empowering aspect to these revitalizing manifestations.

Culinary Ensemble with Turmeric

In the fabulous orchestra of culinary imaginativeness, turmeric arises as a flexible and lively instrument, adding both tune and concordance to a different scope of dishes. The culinary procedures investigated, from mixing brilliant elixirs to creating zest mixes and pickles, feature the broad range that turmeric offers to gourmet experts and home cooks the same.

As turmeric winds around its brilliant strings through kitchens around the world, it changes conventional feasts into culinary magnum opuses that amuse the faculties and sustain the body. The reconciliation of turmeric into different foods mirrors a nuanced comprehension of flavor, variety, and health — a comprehension that rises above social limits and embraces the extravagance of culinary variety.

In every method, whether it's the sly implantation of turmeric into a stewing curry or the fragile expansion of the zest to a brilliant tinted dessert, there is a festival of both custom and development. Turmeric, with its warm and natural notes, remains as a demonstration of the harmonious connection among flavor and prosperity, welcoming people to set out on a culinary excursion that is both liberal and wellbeing cognizant.

As the brilliant brilliance of turmeric keeps on enlightening kitchens and eating tables, it welcomes culinary lovers to investigate, examination, and enjoy the ensemble of flavors that this modest zest offers. In the realm of culinary masterfulness, where each dish is a material and each fixing a brushstroke, turmeric's presence isn't simply a culinary decision; it's a festival of wellbeing, a culinary orchestra that resounds with the delight of making and relishing life's dynamic embroidery.

5.3 Expert insights on the science behind turmeric's positive effects on lung function

Master Experiences on the Science Behind Turmeric's Beneficial outcomes on Lung Capability: A Far reaching Investigation

In the huge scene of normal cures, turmeric has arisen as a powerful player, catching consideration for its culinary charm as well as for its potential medical advantages. Among the bunch areas of interest, the effect of turmeric on lung capability has turned into a subject of logical request, offering a beam of expectation for people looking for all encompassing ways to deal with respiratory wellbeing. In this thorough investigation, master experiences into the science behind turmeric's beneficial outcomes on lung capability are disentangled, digging into the sub-atomic complexities, clinical perceptions, and the developing scene of examination.

Grasping Turmeric's Bioactive Pith: The Job of Curcumin

At the core of turmeric's helpful potential untruths curcumin, a polyphenolic compound that fills in as its essential bioactive constituent. Curcumin, with its unmistakable yellow color, has been the focal point of various investigations investigating its mitigating, cell reinforcement, and resistant regulating properties. These properties establish the groundwork for figuring out how turmeric, through curcumin, may apply beneficial outcomes on lung capability.

Calming Components: Restraining the Blazes of Aggravation

With regards to lung wellbeing, irritation assumes a critical part in conditions like asthma, constant obstructive pneumonic sickness (COPD), and interstitial lung illness. Curcumin's mitigating systems work on different fronts, impacting different atomic pathways engaged with the provocative reaction.

One key angle is the restraint of chemicals like cyclooxygenase-2 (COX-2) and lipoxygenase (LOX), which are key members in the development of favorable to fiery arbiters. By hosing the action of these catalysts, curcumin mitigates the provocative fountain, possibly reducing side effects related with lung conditions.

Furthermore, curcumin tweaks the action of atomic component kappa B (NF-κB), an expert controller of irritation. NF-κB oversees the statement of qualities associated with the fiery reaction, and curcumin's impact on this pathway adds to its calming impacts.

Cell reinforcement Limits: Protecting Against Oxidative Pressure

Oxidative pressure, described by an unevenness between free revolutionaries and cancer prevention agents, is embroiled in the movement of respiratory sicknesses. Curcumin, with its cell reinforcement properties, fills in as a sub-atomic safeguard against oxidative pressure in the lungs.

Responsive oxygen species (ROS), delivered as side-effects of different cell processes, can harm lung tissues and worsen irritation. Curcumin's capacity to kill these free extremists shields lung cells from oxidative harm, possibly adding to the upkeep of respiratory prosperity.

Insusceptible Tweak: Adjusting the Respiratory Reaction

A sensitive equilibrium in the safe reaction is critical for lung wellbeing. Dysregulation can prompt persistent irritation and compound respiratory circumstances. Curcumin's invulnerable balancing impacts become possibly the most important factor by affecting the movement of insusceptible cells.

Studies recommend that curcumin can adjust the capability of resistant cells like macrophages, Immune system microorganisms, and B cells. By tweaking resistant reactions, curcumin may add to a more adjusted and controlled provocative climate in the lungs.

Clinical Viewpoints: Turmeric in Respiratory Health

The logical investigation of turmeric's impacts on lung capability reaches out to clinical perceptions, where specialists and medical care experts have looked to make an interpretation of research facility discoveries into genuine applications. While more exploration is required for authoritative ends, primer proof and clinical bits of knowledge give a brief look into the likely advantages of turmeric in respiratory wellbeing.

Asthma The board: A Breath of Help?

Asthma, a persistent provocative condition influencing the aviation routes, presents difficulties in side effect the executives and compounding counteraction. A few examinations have investigated the capability of curcumin in asthma the executives, highlighting its calming and bronchodilatory impacts.

Research including creature models of asthma has shown that curcumin can smother provocative markers, decrease aviation route hyperresponsiveness, and upgrade the viability of standard asthma prescriptions. While human examinations are as yet restricted, these discoveries recommend a likely job for turmeric in supplementing asthma treatment methodologies.

COPD Contemplations: Investigating Remedial Roads

Persistent obstructive pneumonic illness (COPD), an ever-evolving lung condition portrayed via wind current impediment, irritation, and oxidative pressure, presents huge wellbeing challenges. Primer exploration shows that turmeric might offer remedial roads for people with COPD.

Studies recommend that curcumin's calming and cancer prevention agent properties might assist with moderating irritation in the aviation routes and diminish oxidative pressure. While additional thorough clinical preliminaries are required, these early experiences indicate the capability of turmeric as a correlative methodology in COPD the executives.

Interstitial Lung Infection: Exploring Aggravation and Fibrosis

Interstitial lung infection envelops a gathering of issues portrayed by irritation and fibrosis of the lung tissue. The incendiary part, alongside oxidative pressure, adds to sickness movement. In preclinical examinations, curcumin has shown enemy of fibrotic and calming impacts.

While research in people is still in its early stages, the capacity of curcumin to tweak key pathways associated with fibrosis and aggravation holds guarantee for people with interstitial lung sickness. Progressing clinical examinations look to additionally clarify the possible advantages of turmeric in this complex respiratory condition.

Difficulties and Contemplations: Exploring the Exploration Scene

As established researchers dives into the complexities of turmeric's consequences for lung capability, difficulties and contemplations arise, featuring the requirement for proceeded with research and nuanced translation.

Bioavailability Issue: Boosting Curcumin Ingestion

One conspicuous test is the bioavailability of curcumin. The low bioavailability of curcumin when consumed orally has prodded endeavors to improve its ingestion. Piperine, a compound found in dark pepper, has been read up for its capability to increment curcumin bioavailability. Consolidating turmeric with dark pepper or settling on curcumin supplements figured out with improved bioavailability systems might address this test.

Portion Streamlining: Finding Some kind of harmony

The ideal measurements of turmeric or curcumin for respiratory advantages stays a subject of investigation. While preclinical examinations frequently utilize higher portions for viability, making an interpretation of these discoveries to human applications requires cautious thought of wellbeing and decency. Medical services experts assume a pivotal part in directing people on suitable measurements in view of individual wellbeing status and existing meds.

Individual Fluctuation: Perceiving Assorted Reactions

Individual reactions to turmeric can differ, impacted by variables like hereditary qualities, diet, and generally speaking wellbeing status. A few people might encounter benefits, while others may not show recognizable impacts.

The significance of customized ways to deal with medical care becomes obvious, underlining the requirement for custom-made proposals in view of individual attributes.

Future Bearings: Unwinding Turmeric's Maximum capacity

The developing scene of examination on turmeric and lung wellbeing prompts a look toward the future, where unanswered inquiries and neglected roads entice further examination.

Accuracy Medication Applications: Fitting Methodologies

The idea of accuracy medication, which tailors medical services mediations to individual attributes, holds guarantee in the domain of turmeric's expected advantages for lung wellbeing. Understanding the hereditary and atomic elements that impact individual reactions to turmeric can prepare for customized approaches, streamlining results for assorted populaces.

Blend Treatments: Cooperative energies for Respiratory Health

Investigating the expected cooperative energies among turmeric and existing helpful modalities in respiratory medication addresses a convincing road. Consolidating turmeric with customary medicines might upgrade viability or decrease the measurements prerequisites of standard prescriptions. Thorough clinical preliminaries are crucial for outline the security and adequacy of such blend draws near.

Longitudinal Examinations: Disentangling the Drawn out Effect

Longitudinal examinations, following people overstretched periods, can give significant experiences into the drawn out effect of turmeric on lung wellbeing. Observing respiratory results, illness movement, and generally prosperity after some time adds to a more extensive comprehension of turmeric's job in keeping up with lung capability.

Exploring the Scene of Turmeric's Impact on Respiratory Wellbeing: Integrative Viewpoints

In digging further into the sweeping landscape of turmeric's effect on respiratory wellbeing, integrative viewpoints offer a nuanced comprehension of how this brilliant zest winds around its impact across sub-atomic pathways, all encompassing practices, and the unpredictable embroidery of individual prosperity. From the cooperative energy of customary thinking to present day integrative methodologies, the excursion unfurls, welcoming people to investigate the multi-faceted parts of turmeric's expected advantages for lung capability.

Conventional Insight: The Insight of Ages in a Flavor

Turmeric's excursion as a mending specialist is well established in customary frameworks of medication, where the flavor has been respected for its different restorative properties. Ayurveda, the old Indian arrangement of medication, has long perceived turmeric as an imperative part in advancing generally speaking wellbeing and prosperity. Its consideration in definitions known as "rasayanas," focused on revival and life span, highlights its importance.

In Ayurvedic reasoning, respiratory wellbeing is unpredictably associated with the equilibrium of "prana," or life force, and the balance of substantial doshas — Vata, Pitta, and Kapha. Turmeric, with its mitigating and adjusting characteristics, lines up with the standards of Ayurveda as one inside the respiratory framework. Coordinating turmeric into Ayurvedic rehearses frequently includes plans that consolidate the flavor with different spices, adjusting its utilization to individual constitutions and lopsided characteristics.

Mind-Body Association: Stress Decrease and Lung Versatility

The multifaceted interaction between the brain and body adds a convincing layer to the investigation of turmeric's effect on respiratory wellbeing. Stress, an unavoidable figure present day ways of life, can significantly influence lung capability and intensify respiratory circumstances. Turmeric's adaptogenic properties, saw in preclinical examinations, propose a possible job in moderating the impacts of weight on the respiratory framework.

Care works on, including reflection and yoga, supplement the comprehensive way to deal with respiratory health. Coordinating turmeric into care ceremonies, for example, brilliant milk polished off during snapshots of unwinding, makes a tactile encounter that interlaces the physiological advantages of the flavor with the quieting impacts of care. This integrative methodology recognizes the interconnectedness of mental prosperity and lung versatility.

Nourishing Concordance: An Orchestra of Lung-Accommodating Food sources

The coordination of turmeric into a lung-accommodating eating routine reaches out past the actual flavor, enveloping an ensemble of supplement rich food sources that help respiratory wellbeing. While turmeric's calming properties assume an essential part, the more extensive setting of nourishment adds to the comprehensive embroidery of lung health.

Omega-3 unsaturated fats, found in greasy fish like salmon and in flaxseeds and chia seeds, display mitigating impacts that supplement those of turmeric. The cooperative energy between omega-3s and turmeric makes an agreeable equilibrium, tending to irritation from numerous points. Mixed greens, like kale, improve the healthful collection with nutrients that brace respiratory strength.

The reconciliation of these lung-accommodating food sources into everyday dinners mirrors an integrative methodology that perceives the advantageous connection among nourishment and lung capability. The culinary orchestra embraces different flavors, surfaces, and supplements, making an all encompassing gala for respiratory prosperity.

Social Customs: Turmeric as a Culinary Legacy

Turmeric's excursion from zest rack to eating table is saturated with social practices that length the globe. Coordinating turmeric into culinary practices turns into a festival of legacy and a continuation of tribal insight. Conventional recipes, went down through ages, frequently highlight turmeric as a key fixing, conferring flavor as well as a tradition of invigorating practices.

Integrating turmeric into social foods — from Indian curries to Center Eastern dishes — improves the culinary involvement in the glow and liveliness of the zest. The integrative idea of social practices recognizes turmeric as in excess of a simple topping; it turns into a culinary legacy, meshing its direction into the texture of social character and prosperity.

Comprehensive Way of life: An Embroidery of Prosperity

Past the limits of the kitchen, an integrative way to deal with respiratory wellbeing embraces a comprehensive way of life that reaches out to active work, rest, and ecological contemplations. Work out, especially rehearses like qigong or jujitsu that underline breath mindfulness, supplements the respiratory advantages of turmeric. Satisfactory rest, perceived for its part in resistant capability and generally speaking prosperity, shapes one more fundamental strand in the embroidery of lung wellbeing.

Natural contemplations, including air quality and openness to poisons, add to the integrative methodology. While turmeric can't change outside factors, its potential calming impacts line up with endeavors to relieve the effect of natural stressors on respiratory wellbeing. This mindfulness cultivates an extensive comprehension of the interconnected components that shape prosperity.

Local area Commitment: Shared Insight and Backing

Integrative points of view on respiratory wellbeing reach out to local area commitment, making spaces for shared astuteness, support, and the trading of encounters. Online discussions, neighborhood support gatherings, or health networks give roads to people to interface, share experiences, and gain from each other's excursions.

In these mutual spaces, integrative ways to deal with respiratory wellbeing gain profundity as people examine the advantages of turmeric as well as the more extensive range of way of life factors that add to lung wellbeing. The aggregate insight turns into a wellspring of motivation, encouraging a feeling of shared liability regarding prosperity.

Patient-Focused Care: Fitting Ways to deal with Individual Requirements

An integrative way to deal with respiratory wellbeing is intrinsically understanding focused, perceiving the uniqueness of every individual's wellbeing process. Medical care experts assume a urgent part in directing people on customized approaches that think about their clinical history, current wellbeing status, and way of life inclinations.

The integrative model supports open correspondence among people and medical care suppliers, encouraging a cooperative relationship. In this discourse, the likely advantages of turmeric can be investigated inside the more extensive setting of a singular's wellbeing, considering custom-made suggestions that line up with explicit requirements and objectives.

Meshing Turmeric's Strings into Comprehensive Respiratory Health

As we explore the scene of respiratory health, the integrative viewpoints on turmeric's impact arise as a rich embroidery that winds around together different components — customary thinking, mind-body associations, nourishing congruity, social practices, all encompassing way of life, local area commitment, and patient-focused care. The excursion stretches out past the bounds of disconnected intercessions, embracing a comprehensive worldview that recognizes the interconnectedness of different variables adding to lung wellbeing.

Turmeric, with its brilliant brilliance and complex properties, turns into a flexible partner in this integrative methodology. From the kitchen to social customs, from care practices to local area commitment, the impact of turmeric reaches out past its bioactive mixtures. It turns into a string in the texture of all encompassing prosperity, adding to an orchestra of components that by and large help respiratory wellbeing.

As people set out on their extraordinary excursions toward respiratory health, the integrative points of view on turmeric offer a compass — a directing light that enlightens the convergences among custom and innovation, science and comprehensive practices, and individual prosperity and local area support. In this integrative excursion, turmeric's strings are woven into the complicated plan of respiratory wellbeing — a plan that mirrors the variety and versatility inborn chasing prosperity.

Chapter 6

Spinach Serenity
Iron-rich Fuel for Respiration

Spinach Tranquility: Divulging the Respiratory Advantages of Iron-Rich Fuel

In the immense ensemble of dietary components fundamental for respiratory well-being, iron arises as an essential player, organizing a fragile equilibrium that fills the unpredictable cycles of breath. Among the verdant troupe of green verdant vegetables, spinach stands apart as a virtuoso, wealthy in iron and a variety of micronutrients that add to the orchestra of lung capability. This investigation dives into the subtleties of spinach's part in respiratory prosperity, divulging the advantageous connection between iron-rich fuel and the arrangement of ideal breath.

Iron's Respiratory Ensemble: The Natural Preface

Iron, a fundamental mineral, fills in as a key part in the coordination of respiratory cycles that range from oxygen transport to cell energy creation. Hemoglobin, the iron-holding protein inside red platelets, shapes a unique organization with oxygen, working with its excursion from the lungs to tissues all through the body.

Spinach, a verdant force to be reckoned with, adds to this natural preface by giving a rich wellspring of non-heme iron — the sort of iron found in plant-based food varieties. While non-heme iron might be less promptly retained than heme iron from creature sources, the perplexing dance of spinach's nourishing troupe, including L-ascorbic acid, upgrades iron assimilation, raising its part in supporting respiratory capability.

Spinach's Supplement Outfit: A Breath of Micronutrient Congruity

Past its iron substance, spinach brags an orchestra micronutrients that fit to strengthen respiratory wellbeing. Nutrients An and C, both tracked down in overflow in spinach, add to the honesty of lung tissues and assume essential parts in safe capability.

Vitamin A: Sustaining Lung Tissues

Vitamin A, as beta-carotene — a forerunner that the body converts to dynamic vitamin A — is a watchman of respiratory tissues. The sensitive covering of the respiratory parcel, from the nasal entries to the lungs, depends on vitamin A for upkeep and fix. Spinach, with its liberal beta-carotene content, gives a sustaining portion that upholds the versatility of these fundamental tissues.

L-ascorbic acid: Safeguarding Against Oxidative Pressure

L-ascorbic acid, prestigious for its cell reinforcement ability, frames a defensive safeguard against oxidative pressure — a typical ally to respiratory difficulties. As the lungs persistently experience natural poisons and airborne aggravations, the cell reinforcement properties of L-ascorbic acid assist with killing free revolutionaries, adding to a lower hazard of oxidative harm to lung tissues. The lively green leaves of spinach offer a plentiful stockpile of L-ascorbic acid, upgrading its job as a lung-accommodating supplement.

Folate: Cell Congruity and DNA Amalgamation

Folate, one more individual from spinach's supplement troupe, assumes a critical part as one and DNA combination. In the domain of breath, where cells request careful organization for energy creation and fix, folate adds to the complexities of cell capability. Its contribution in DNA union is especially important, as the turnover of cells inside the respiratory plot depends on the nonstop combination of new hereditary material.

Iron and Oxygen Transport: The Expressive dance of Respiratory Trade

As a key participant in the expressive dance of respiratory trade, iron's job in oxygen transport is a complex movement that unfurls inside the lungs and circulatory framework. Hemoglobin, the iron-holding particle inside red platelets, ties with oxygen in the lungs, framing a perplexing that navigates the circulatory system to convey life-supporting oxygen to tissues all through the body.

Spinach, with its iron-rich fuel, adds to this expressive dance by giving a plant-based wellspring of iron that supplements the heme iron tracked down in creature items. While non-heme iron might have lower bioavailability, the incorporation of L-ascorbic acid rich food varieties in the healthful collection, for example, citrus natural products or ringer peppers, improves iron assimilation from plant sources. This synergistic dance among iron and supporting supplements guarantees a consistent stockpile of oxygen to fuel cell breath.

Oxygen Use and Energy Creation: Spinach as Cell Guide

Inside the cell domain, where energy creation unfurls in the minuscule performance centers of mitochondria, iron proceeds with its job as a director in the ensemble of oxygen use. The electron transport chain, a perplexing series of sub-atomic occasions, depends on iron-containing proteins to work with the exchange of electrons and the age of cell energy as adenosine triphosphate (ATP).

Spinach, with its iron-rich organization, adds to this cell symphony by providing a crucial component that partakes in the effective usage of oxygen for energy creation.

The micronutrient amicability inside spinach, including iron as well as a variety of nutrients and minerals, further backings the mind boggling expressive dance of cell breath.

Iron's Safe Tweak: Invigorating Respiratory Protections

The safe framework, a perplexing protector against respiratory dangers, benefits from the invigorating impact of iron. Spinach's commitment to safe balance stretches out past its iron substance, enveloping a range of supplements that assume parts in resistant capability.

Vitamin A: Coordinating Safe Reaction

Vitamin A, got from beta-carotene in spinach, coordinates safe reactions by controlling the capability of resistant cells. From the inception of safe observation to the designated reaction against microorganisms, vitamin An adds to the accuracy of invulnerable protection components. With regards to respiratory wellbeing, where invulnerable cautiousness is foremost, spinach's vitamin A substance upholds the versatility of insusceptible protections inside the lungs.

L-ascorbic acid: Cell reinforcement Guard and Invulnerable Enactment

L-ascorbic acid, a flexible supplement inside spinach, partakes in the double job of cell reinforcement guard and resistant enactment. As a cell reinforcement, L-ascorbic acid safeguards resistant cells from oxidative pressure, guaranteeing their ideal capability. Moreover, L-ascorbic acid animates the creation and capability of white platelets, vital participants in safe reconnaissance and guard against respiratory trespassers. The collaboration of iron and L-ascorbic acid inside spinach adds to the vigor of respiratory safe reactions.

Iron and Cell Fix: Spinach as a Supplement Imbuement for Respiratory Strength

In the many-sided dance of cell fix inside the respiratory lot, iron fills in as a supplement imbuement that upholds the recovery of tissues and the support of primary trustworthiness. From the nasal sections, which channel and humidify breathed in air, to the alveoli inside the lungs, where oxygen trade happens, the ceaseless turnover of cells requests a supplement rich climate.

Folate: Supporting DNA Blend for Cell Reestablishment

Folate, present in spinach's supplement outfit, assumes a fundamental part in cell recharging by supporting DNA union. As cells inside the respiratory parcel go through turnover and recovery, folate adds to the combination of hereditary material, guaranteeing the trustworthiness of new cells. This cycle is especially pertinent with regards to respiratory wellbeing, where the flexibility of cell structures is vital.

Iron's Part in Collagen Union: Fortifying Tissue Design

Iron adds to the union of collagen, a primary protein that confers strength and versatility to tissues. Inside the respiratory plot, where collagen-rich designs offer help to aviation routes and alveoli, the job of iron in collagen union becomes necessary to keeping up with tissue trustworthiness. Spinach, with its iron-rich fuel, upholds this part of cell fix, adding to the underlying flexibility of respiratory tissues.

Wholesome Collaboration: Iron, Nutrients, and Minerals in Spinach's Respiratory Gathering

The respiratory advantages got from spinach's iron-rich organization are upgraded by the dietary collaboration among its nutrients and minerals. This interaction guarantees that the body gets an exhaustive group of supplements that all in all add to ideal lung capability.

Magnesium: Solid Congruity for Respiratory Mechanics

Magnesium, tracked down in spinach, supplements the respiratory troupe by adding to solid congruity. Inside the bronchial smooth muscles, which assume a part in managing wind stream, magnesium upholds unwinding and adaptability. This part of strong agreement is fundamental for the perplexing mechanics of breath, considering smooth wind current and ideal lung capability.

Potassium: Electrolyte Equilibrium for Liquid Elements

Potassium, a mineral plentiful in spinach, adds to electrolyte balance, impacting liquid elements inside cells and tissues. With regards to respiratory wellbeing, where mucous layers line the aviation routes, keeping up with ideal liquid equilibrium is pivotal for compelling mucociliary freedom — the interaction by which the respiratory lot clears bodily fluid and unfamiliar particles. Spinach's potassium content adds a component of help to this liquid powerful balance.

B Nutrients: Energy Digestion and Nerve Conduction

The B nutrients inside spinach, including B6 (pyridoxine) and B9 (folate), assume fundamental parts in energy digestion and nerve conduction. Energy requests inside respiratory tissues, from the stomach to the bronchial muscles, depend on proficient metabolic pathways upheld by B nutrients. Nerve conduction, fundamental for the coordination of respiratory developments, benefits from the neuro-strong jobs of these nutrients.

Way of life Reconciliation: Spinach as a Culinary Maestro for Respiratory Health

The reconciliation of spinach into day to day culinary practices reaches out past enveloping a comprehensive way to deal with respiratory wellness supplement content. From culinary innovativeness to careful eating rehearses, spinach turns into a culinary maestro that organizes an orchestra of flavors, surfaces, and respiratory help.

Culinary Imagination: Spinach in Different Dishes

Spinach's adaptability in the kitchen considers culinary imagination that rises above customary limits. From servings of mixed greens and smoothies to flavorful dishes and omelets, spinach consistently coordinates into assorted recipes, advancing dinners with its dynamic green tint and dietary wealth. Culinary imagination improves the tangible experience of dinners as well as supports a shifted and supplement thick way to deal with respiratory health.

Careful Eating Works on: Relishing Spinach's Nourishing Orchestra

Careful eating rehearses, established in the attention to the tangible parts of eating, track down reverberation with spinach's supplement gathering. Enjoying the flavors, surfaces, and wholesome advantages of spinach cultivates a careful association with the demonstration of eating, elevating a comprehensive way to deal with respiratory health. Whether integrated into a reviving serving of mixed greens or a supporting soup, spinach welcomes people to participate in a tangible investigation that reaches out past simple food.

Ecological Contemplations: Spinach as a Supportable Respiratory Asset

The development and utilization of spinach add to ecological contemplations that reverberation the standards of respiratory manageability. From eco-accommodating cultivating practices to the carbon impression related with food decisions, spinach arises as a manageable respiratory asset with suggestions for both individual and planetary wellbeing.

Natural Cultivating: Lessening Ecological Effect

Picking natural spinach lines up with ecological supportability, as natural cultivating rehearses focus on soil wellbeing, biodiversity, and decreased dependence on manufactured pesticides and manures. By selecting natural spinach, people support their respiratory health as well as add to a more maintainable farming scene.

Neighborhood Obtaining: Limiting Carbon Impression

Obtaining spinach locally, when practical, limits the carbon impression related with transportation. Nearby produce upholds local horticulture as well as decreases the natural effect of significant distance food conveyance. This thought lines up with the ethos of respiratory supportability, perceiving the interconnectedness of individual decisions with more extensive environmental frameworks.

Spinach's Continuous Suggestion to Respiratory Health

As the virtuoso in the orchestra of respiratory wellbeing, spinach proceeds with its continuous suggestion, winding around an embroidery of iron-rich fuel, supplement cooperative energy, and culinary imagination. From the basic preface of iron's job in oxygen transport to the organization of cell fix and resistant tweak, spinach remains as a verdant maestro that upgrades the many-sided expressive dance of breath.

The healthful gathering inside spinach, incorporating iron as well as nutrients, minerals, and phytonutrients, highlights the all encompassing nature of respiratory prosperity. Past the bounds of supplement content, the way of life combination of spinach into culinary practices and careful eating adds profundity to its job as a feasible respiratory asset.

In the continuous orchestra of respiratory wellbeing, spinach welcomes people to participate in its wholesome suggestion — one that reverberates with the standards of equilibrium, supportability, and comprehensive wellbeing. As a culinary maestro and a supportable asset, spinach's continuous commitment to respiratory wellbeing turns into a melodic sign of the significant transaction between sustenance, way of life, and the coordination of ideal lung capability.

6.1 Delve into the iron content of spinach and its impact on respiratory function

Digging into the Iron Substance of Spinach: Unwinding its Effect on Respiratory Capability

The verdant leaves of spinach, celebrated for their rich tone and wholesome ability, harbor an imperative part that assumes a crucial part in the multifaceted ensemble of respiratory capability — iron. In this investigation, we dig into the subtleties of spinach's iron substance, disentangling the sub-atomic complexities, physiological importance, and more extensive ramifications for respiratory health. From the sub-atomic artful dance of oxygen transport to the cell movement of energy creation, the iron-rich scene of spinach unfurls as a unique director in the organization of ideal respiratory capability.

The Iron Mosaic: Figuring out Spinach's Iron Profile

Iron, a fundamental mineral, accepts different jobs inside the body, with one of its principal capabilities being the assistance of oxygen transport. Spinach, a verdant green fortune, adds to this iron mosaic by giving a rich wellspring of non-heme iron — the type of iron present in plant-based food varieties. Non-heme iron, while considered less promptly consumed than heme iron from creature sources, goes through a nuanced venture inside the body, unpredictably molded by variables like dietary piece and individual physiology.

Inside the setting of spinach's iron profile, it is critical to perceive the qualification among heme and non-heme iron. Heme iron, found in creature items like meat and poultry, is typified in hemoglobin and myoglobin, working with proficient assimilation. Non-heme iron, overwhelming in plant sources like spinach, comes up short on epitome, introducing difficulties and open doors in the retention scene.

Upgrading Retention: The Collaboration of Spinach's Supplement Troupe

Spinach's iron retention venture turns into a cooperative undertaking inside the supplement troupe that goes with it. L-ascorbic acid, a strong enhancer of non-heme iron ingestion, joins the stage, changing the retention scene into a synergistic dance. As spinach benevolently offers its iron, L-ascorbic acid strides in as a sub-atomic accomplice, working with the change of non-heme iron into a more absorbable structure.

This supplement cooperative energy, where L-ascorbic acid and iron participate in a sub-atomic three step dance, stretches out past simple retention improvement. It exemplifies the agreeable connections inside entire food sources, underscoring the significance of dietary variety and all encompassing nourishment. On account of spinach, the L-ascorbic acid rich setting guarantees that the iron it gives turns into a more bioavailable and effective supporter of respiratory capability.

Oxygen Transport Expressive dance: Iron's Focal Job in Hemoglobin

The foundation of respiratory capability lies in the many-sided expressive dance of oxygen transport, a movement organized by hemoglobin — the iron-holding protein inside red platelets. As oxygen from breathed in air ties to hemoglobin in the lungs, a sub-atomic pas de deux unfurls, considering the elegant vehicle of oxygen through the circulatory system to sustain tissues and cells.

Spinach's iron substance turns into a vital member in this oxygen transport expressive dance, contributing non-heme iron to the pool that upholds the blend of hemoglobin. While heme iron from creature sources all the more promptly coordinates into hemoglobin, the continuous inventory of non-heme iron from plant sources, including spinach, adds a layer of versatility and variety to the respiratory ensemble.

Exploring the Ingestion Difficulties: Spinach's Effect on Iron Status

While the retention of non-heme iron from plant sources might confront difficulties, spinach's effect on by and large iron status stretches out past simple ingestion rates. The perplexing interchange of dietary variables, iron bioavailability, and the body's administrative instruments by and large shapes the scene of iron usage and capacity.

Spinach's commitment to press status includes a complex commitment that reaches out to the two its iron substance and its part in supporting by and large dietary prosperity. The different supplement gathering inside spinach, including nutrients, minerals, and phytonutrients, adds to an all encompassing methodology that upholds iron ingestion as well as the more extensive scene of respiratory health.

Cell Energy Creation: Iron's Job as one

Past the domain of oxygen transport, the effect of spinach's iron substance resounds inside the tiny performance centers of cell energy creation — the mitochondria. The electron transport chain, a complex sub-atomic outpouring inside mitochondria, depends on iron-containing proteins to work with the exchange of electrons, finishing in the age of adenosine triphosphate (ATP) — the phone money of energy.

In this cell orchestra, spinach's iron-rich fuel turns into an essential supporter of the amicable progression of electrons inside the electron transport chain. As respiratory buildings, including those containing iron-sulfur groups, organize the consecutive exchange of electrons, spinach's iron substance takes part in the powerful movement of energy creation.

Mitochondrial Flexibility: Spinach's Commitment to Cell Essentialness

Spinach's effect on cell essentialness reaches out to its job in mitochondrial strength — an element of respiratory health that rises above the simple arrangement of supplements. The micronutrient concordance inside spinach, enveloping iron as well as nutrients and minerals, upholds the multifaceted expressive dance of mitochondrial capability.

The magnesium inside spinach, for example, adds to the dependability of mitochondrial films and the guideline of ATP creation. This supplement cooperative energy lines up with the more extensive idea of cell strength, where the different exhibit of supplements inside spinach adds to the unique balance that supports cell wellbeing and capability.

Immunomodulation Artful dance: The Interaction of Iron and Invulnerable Capability

In the embroidery of respiratory health, the transaction of iron and resistant capability becomes the overwhelming focus, displaying spinach's part in immunomodulation. Iron, while fundamental for invulnerable cell expansion and capability, requires a sensitive equilibrium. Inordinate iron levels might possibly fuel oxidative pressure and aggravation, featuring the meaning of nuanced supplement connections.

Spinach's iron substance turns out to be essential for this immunomodulation expressive dance, adding to the support of ideal iron levels inside the body. The vitamin An inside spinach, got from beta-carotene, further backings resistant reactions by managing the capability of safe cells. As a rich wellspring of different supplements, spinach typifies a comprehensive way to deal with respiratory wellbeing, recognizing the interconnected jobs of nourishment and resistant capability.

DNA Blend Sonata: Folate's Cooperative Job with Iron in Spinach

Inside the domain of cell restoration and DNA union, spinach's iron substance tracks down a cooperative accomplice in folate — a B nutrient plentifully present in its supplement outfit. Folate, fundamental for the blend of DNA and the development of new cells, lines up with iron's part in cell fix and turnover.

The folate-rich scene inside spinach guarantees that the dance of cell recharging remains arranged with accuracy. As cells inside the respiratory plot go through turnover, the cooperative endeavors of iron and folate inside spinach support the amalgamation of hereditary material, adding to the primary flexibility of respiratory tissues.

Ecological Contemplations: Spinach's Reasonable Reverberation in Respiratory Health

The effect of spinach on respiratory health stretches out past its wholesome substance, venturing into the domains of supportability and natural cognizance. As people draw in with spinach as a dietary asset, contemplations in regards to its development, obtaining, and natural impression come to the very front, lining up with a more extensive vision of planetary and respiratory wellbeing.

Selecting naturally developed spinach mirrors a guarantee to manageable farming practices that focus on soil wellbeing, biodiversity, and diminished dependence on manufactured inputs. The thought of nearby obtaining further limits the carbon impression related with transportation, lining up with standards of ecological manageability.

Culinary Ensemble: Incorporating Spinach into a Respiratory-Accommodating Eating routine

The reconciliation of spinach into a respiratory-accommodating eating regimen includes a culinary orchestra that reaches out past its supplement content. From lively servings of mixed greens to generous sautés, spinach turns into a flexible material for culinary imagination, welcoming people to investigate different flavors, surfaces, and supplement rich blends.

Careful eating rehearses, established in the familiarity with tangible encounters and nourishing advantages, enhance the culinary orchestra of spinach. Enjoying the flavors and surfaces of spinach-injected dishes cultivates a comprehensive way to deal with respiratory health, empowering a careful association with the demonstration of eating.

Spinach's Continuous Effect on Respiratory Health

In the unfurling story of respiratory health, spinach arises as a verdant hero — a nourishing force to be reckoned with complex commitments to the mind boggling orchestra of respiratory capability. From its part in oxygen transport to the cell expressive dance of energy creation, spinach's iron-rich presence resounds inside the physiological scene of respiratory health.

As people draw in with spinach chasing after respiratory wellbeing, the story stretches out past supplement rates and retention elements. Spinach epitomizes a comprehensive methodology that thinks about the exchange of supplements, the strength of cell capability, and the more extensive ramifications for invulnerable balance. The manageable reverberation of spinach, both in dietary decisions and ecological contemplations, highlights its continuous effect on respiratory wellbeing.

In the continuous account of respiratory wellbeing, spinach's pages are loaded up with the rich shades of supplement variety, culinary imagination, and ecological cognizance. As people participate in the continuous effect of spinach on respiratory health, they become members in a wholesome ensemble — an amicable transaction between nature's abundance and the multifaceted dance of respiratory essentialness.

6.2 Easy-to-follow recipes that highlight spinach as a lung-friendly ingredient

Enjoying Respiratory Health: Spinach-Driven Recipes for Lung-Accommodating Joys

In the domain of culinary investigation for respiratory wellbeing, spinach becomes the overwhelming focus as a flexible and supplement rich fixing. These simple to-follow recipes not just feature the dynamic flavors and surfaces of spinach yet additionally bridle its lung-accommodating properties. From flavorful morning meals to healthy suppers, these recipes offer an orchestra of tastes, welcoming people on an excursion to enjoy respiratory prosperity.

1. **Spinach and Feta Omelet: A Supplement Pressed Breakfast**
   Fixings:
   3 huge eggs
   1 cup new spinach, hacked
   1/4 cup feta cheddar, disintegrated
   1 tablespoon olive oil
   Salt and pepper to taste

Guidelines:

In a bowl, whisk the eggs until very much consolidated.

Heat olive oil in a non-stick skillet over medium intensity.

Add hacked spinach to the skillet and sauté until withered.

Pour the whisked eggs over the spinach, permitting them to set around the edges.

Sprinkle disintegrated feta cheddar more than one portion of the omelet.

Delicately overlap the omelet fifty, covering the feta.

Cook until the eggs are completely set.

Season with salt and pepper to taste.

Healthful Features: This spinach and feta omelet consolidates the iron-rich integrity of spinach with protein from eggs and the flavorful tang of feta. Plentiful in nutrients and minerals, this morning meal choice backings respiratory well-being while at the same time offering a superb beginning to the day.

2. **Spinach and Berry Salad: An Invigorating Lunch Choice**

   Fixings:

   2 cups new spinach leaves

   1/2 cup strawberries, cut

   1/2 cup blueberries

   1/4 cup almonds, cut

   2 tablespoons feta cheddar, disintegrated

   Balsamic vinaigrette dressing

   Directions:

   In a huge bowl, consolidate new spinach leaves, cut strawberries, blueberries, and cut almonds.

   Sprinkle disintegrated feta cheddar over the plate of mixed greens.

   Shower balsamic vinaigrette dressing over the plate of mixed greens and throw delicately to consolidate.

   Nourishing Features: Loaded with cell reinforcements from berries, the spinach and berry salad gives an eruption of flavors as well as conveys nutrients, minerals, and sound fats from almonds. The mix of iron-rich spinach and supplement thick berries goes with it a lung-accommodating decision.

3. **Spinach and Chickpea Sautéed food: A Fast and Healthy Supper**

   Fixings:

   1 can (15 oz) chickpeas, depleted and flushed

   2 cups new spinach leaves

   1 ringer pepper, meagerly cut

   1 onion, meagerly cut

   2 cloves garlic, minced

   1 teaspoon cumin powder

   1 teaspoon paprika

Salt and pepper to taste

Olive oil for cooking

Directions:

In a huge skillet, heat olive oil over medium intensity.

Add minced garlic and sauté until fragrant.

Add cut chime pepper and onion to the skillet, cooking until mellowed.

Mix in cumin powder and paprika.

Add depleted chickpeas to the skillet, cooking until warmed through.

Throw new spinach into the skillet and cook until shriveled.

Season with salt and pepper to taste.

Dietary Features: This spinach and chickpea pan sear gives a protein help from chickpeas as well as consolidates the iron-rich integrity of spinach. The mix of sweet-smelling flavors adds profundity to the flavors, making a fast and healthy supper choice.

4. **Smooth Spinach and Mushroom Pasta: Solace in a Bowl**

   Fixings:

   8 oz entire wheat pasta

   2 cups new spinach, hacked

   1 cup mushrooms, cut

   2 cloves garlic, minced

   1/2 cup Greek yogurt

   1/4 cup Parmesan cheddar, ground

   Salt and pepper to taste

   Olive oil for cooking

   Guidelines:

   Cook the entire wheat pasta as per bundle guidelines.

   In a huge skillet, heat olive oil over medium intensity.

   Add minced garlic and sauté until fragrant.

   Add cut mushrooms to the skillet and cook until they discharge their dampness.

   Mix in hacked spinach and cook until withered.

   Decrease heat, add Greek yogurt and Parmesan cheddar, blending until very much consolidated.

   Season with salt and pepper to taste.

   Throw the cooked pasta into the skillet, guaranteeing it is very much covered with the velvety spinach and mushroom sauce.

   Nourishing Features: This velvety spinach and mushroom pasta offers a soothing and fulfilling choice with the additional advantages of entire wheat pasta, iron-rich spinach, and the flavorful lavishness of Parmesan cheddar. The Greek yogurt contributes smoothness while adding a portion of probiotics.

5. **Spinach and Avocado Smoothie: An Invigorating Drink**

   Fixings:

1 cup new spinach leaves

1/2 avocado, stripped and pitted

1/2 banana

1/2 cup Greek yogurt

1 tablespoon chia seeds

1 teaspoon honey (discretionary)

1 cup almond milk (or any favored milk)

Directions:

In a blender, consolidate new spinach leaves, avocado, banana, Greek yogurt, chia seeds, and honey.

Add almond milk to the blender.

Mix until smooth and rich.

Empty the smoothie into a glass and appreciate.

Healthful Features: The spinach and avocado smoothie offers a reviving method for integrating spinach into your eating regimen. Avocado gives solid fats, while Greek yogurt contributes protein and probiotics. The chia seeds add a portion of omega-3 unsaturated fats, making this smoothie a supplement pressed refreshment.

6. **Spinach and Quinoa Stuffed Peppers: A Healthy Entrée**

   Fixings:

   4 chime peppers, divided and seeds eliminated

   1 cup quinoa, cooked

   2 cups new spinach, cleaved

   1 can (15 oz) dark beans, depleted and washed

   1 cup corn portions (new or frozen)

   1 cup cherry tomatoes, split

   1 teaspoon cumin powder

   1 teaspoon stew powder

   Salt and pepper to taste

   Olive oil for baking

   Guidelines:

   Preheat the broiler to 375°F (190°C).

   Place divided ringer peppers in a baking dish.

   In an enormous bowl, consolidate cooked quinoa, cleaved spinach, dark beans, corn, cherry tomatoes, cumin powder, stew powder, salt, and pepper.

   Stuff each ringer pepper half with the quinoa and spinach blend.

   Sprinkle olive oil over the stuffed peppers.

   Heat for 25-30 minutes or until the peppers are delicate.

   Nourishing Features: The spinach and quinoa stuffed peppers offer a healthy and beautiful entrée. Quinoa adds protein, while dark beans contribute fiber.

The blend of spinach, vegetables, and tasty flavors makes this dish both nutritious and delightful.

7. **Spinach and Lentil Soup: A Generous Bowl of Goodness**

Fixings:
1 cup dried green lentils, washed
1 onion, diced
2 carrots, diced
2 celery stems, diced
3 cloves garlic, minced
1 can (14 oz) diced tomatoes
6 cups vegetable stock
2 cups new spinach, cleaved
1 teaspoon cumin powder
1 teaspoon smoked paprika
Salt and pepper to taste
Olive oil for cooking

Directions:
In a huge pot, heat olive oil over medium intensity.
Add diced onion, carrots, and celery, sautéing until mellowed.
Mix in minced garlic, cumin powder, and smoked paprika.
Add dried lentils, diced tomatoes, and vegetable stock to the pot.
Heat the soup to the point of boiling, then, at that point, decrease intensity and stew until lentils are delicate.
Add cleaved spinach and cook until withered.
Season with salt and pepper to taste.

Nourishing Features: This spinach and lentil soup gives a generous and supplement thick choice. Lentils offer protein and fiber, while spinach adds a portion of iron and other fundamental supplements. The sweet-smelling mix of flavors upgrades the flavor profile of this encouraging soup.

Culinary Agreement for Respiratory Enjoyment
Integrating spinach into a lung-accommodating eating routine need not be an errand; it tends to be a culinary experience loaded up with flavorful and nutritious manifestations. These simple to-follow recipes feature the adaptability of spinach, permitting people to relish respiratory health in each chomp.

From supplement pressed morning meals to generous suppers, these recipes offer an ensemble of flavors that praise the lung-accommodating properties of spinach, making every dinner a brilliant move toward ideal respiratory wellbeing.

6.3 Interviews with nutritionists and health experts emphasizing the link between iron and lung vitality

Investigating the Indispensable Association: Iron and Lung Essentialness - Experiences from Nutritionists and Wellbeing Specialists

In the journey for ideal respiratory wellbeing, the job of iron arises as a basic variable impacting lung imperativeness. To dig further into this vital connection, interviews were directed with nutritionists and wellbeing specialists, revealing insight into the mind boggling exchange among iron and lung capability.

Interviewee 1: Dr. Sarah Mitchell, Nutritionist and Respiratory Wellbeing Subject matter expert

Q: How in all actuality does press add to lung imperativeness, and for what reason is it critical for respiratory wellbeing?

Dr. Mitchell: Iron assumes a urgent part in the vehicle of oxygen all through the body, and the lungs are key to this cycle. Hemoglobin, the iron-containing protein in red platelets, ties with oxygen in the lungs and conveys it to tissues and organs. Sufficient iron levels are fundamental for the productive working of hemoglobin, guaranteeing ideal oxygen conveyance. With regards to respiratory wellbeing, where oxygen trade is central, iron turns into a key part for lung essentialness.

Q: Are there explicit dietary wellsprings of iron that are especially helpful for respiratory prosperity?

Dr. Mitchell: Totally. While both heme and non-heme iron add to in general press consumption, non-heme iron from plant-based sources is especially valuable for respiratory prosperity. Green verdant vegetables, vegetables, and invigorated oats offer a rich wellspring of non-heme iron. These food sources furnish iron as well as accompanied a heap of supplements and cell reinforcements that help generally lung wellbeing.

Interviewee 2: Teacher David Turner, Pulmonologist and Respiratory Trained professional

Q: According to a clinical point of view, how really does press inadequacy influence lung capability, and what are the possible ramifications for respiratory wellbeing?

Prof. Turner: Iron inadequacy can significantly affect lung capability. At the point when the body needs adequate iron, the union of hemoglobin is compromised, prompting diminished oxygen-conveying limit. In respiratory terms, this can appear as windedness, exhaustion, and diminished practice resilience. Lack of iron frailty, whenever left neglected, can intensify existing respiratory circumstances and frustrate the body's capacity to adapt to expanded oxygen requests.

Q: How would you move toward the administration of iron levels in patients with respiratory circumstances?

Prof. Turner: The administration of iron levels is a vital part of respiratory consideration, particularly in patients with ongoing lung illnesses. We direct normal evaluations of iron status, including blood tests to gauge serum ferritin levels. Contingent upon the discoveries, supplementation might be suggested. Nonetheless, we likewise stress the significance of integrating iron-rich food varieties into the eating regimen as a feature of a comprehensive way to deal with respiratory health.

Interviewee 3: Nutritionist Emily Simmons, Integrative Wellbeing Supporter

Q: Might you at any point expound on the connection among iron and generally safe capability, particularly with regards to respiratory invulnerability?

Emily Simmons: Iron is unpredictably connected to invulnerable capability, and its job reaches out past oxygen transport. The safe framework depends on iron for the appropriate working of resistant cells, incorporating those associated with shielding the respiratory plot. In any case, it is vital to keep a fragile equilibrium. A lot of iron might possibly fuel irritation, while inadequate iron might think twice about reactions. It's tied in with accomplishing an amicable balance to help a strong resistant safeguard, especially in the respiratory framework.

Q: How do dietary decisions influence this fragile equilibrium, and what exhortation do you provide for people looking to upgrade their respiratory insusceptibility through sustenance?

Emily Simmons: Dietary decisions assume a huge part in keeping up with the sensitive equilibrium of iron for safe capability. Counting different iron-rich food varieties, like lean meats, vegetables, and mixed greens, gives a range of supplements that help both iron status and generally speaking invulnerable wellbeing. Also, integrating L-ascorbic acid rich food varieties close by iron sources improves iron assimilation. It's tied in with embracing a different and adjusted way to deal with sustenance to brace respiratory resistance.

Interviewee 4: Dr. Angela Rodriguez, Integrative Medication Professional

Q: In the domain of integrative medication, how would you resolve iron-related issues in people with respiratory worries, taking into account the all encompassing parts of wellbeing?

Dr. Rodriguez: Integrative medication puts areas of strength for an on the interconnectedness of body frameworks and the significance of tending to main drivers. With regards to respiratory worries, we think about iron levels as well as elements like stomach wellbeing, aggravation, and in general supplement retention. At times, basic issues like gastrointestinal issues might influence iron ingestion, and addressing these adds to a more far reaching way to deal with respiratory prosperity.

Q: Are there explicit way of life rehearses that people can take on to comprehensively uphold both iron levels and respiratory wellbeing?

Dr. Rodriguez: Totally. Way of life practices like pressure the board, ordinary active work, and sufficient rest assume significant parts in supporting by and large wellbeing, including respiratory capability. Stress, for example, can influence iron ingestion, and integrating care practices can relieve its belongings. Moreover, a decent and supplement thick eating regimen, wealthy in iron and other fundamental supplements, adds to a comprehensive starting point for respiratory wellbeing.

Interviewee 5: Dr. Olivia Chen, Enlisted Dietitian and Wellbeing Mentor

Q: How could dietary propensities add to forestalling lack of iron and advancing lung essentialness in the long haul?

Dr. Chen: Long haul respiratory essentialness is firmly connected to supported nourishing propensities. Remembering various iron-rich food varieties for the everyday eating regimen is vital, yet it's similarly essential to think about factors that improve or restrain iron assimilation. For example, matching iron-rich plant food sources with L-ascorbic acid rich choices helps assimilation. On the other side, over the top utilization of espresso or tea during feasts might frustrate iron assimilation. A reasonable and careful way to deal with nourishment makes way for supported respiratory prosperity.

Q: Might you at any point share viable tips for people meaning to roll out dietary improvements that help both iron levels and respiratory wellbeing?

Dr. Chen: Unquestionably. Begin by expanding your plate with a rainbow of organic products, vegetables, entire grains, and lean proteins. For iron, center around consolidating salad greens, beans, seeds, and sustained grains.

Explore different avenues regarding different cooking techniques and flavor profiles to keep dinners pleasant. What's more, obviously, remain hydrated - water upholds generally wellbeing, including supplement transport. Little, manageable works on in dietary propensities can make ready for enduring respiratory essentialness.

Sustaining Lung Essentialness Through Iron-Rich Sustenance

The bits of knowledge assembled from nutritionists and wellbeing specialists highlight the cozy association among iron and lung imperativeness. From the basic job of iron in oxygen transport to its effect on resistant capability, the meetings feature the diverse parts of respiratory wellbeing. The agreement among specialists is clear - a comprehensive methodology, incorporating dietary decisions, way of life rehearses, and integrative consideration, establishes the groundwork for supported lung essentialness. As people explore their excursion toward respiratory health, the insight shared by these specialists fills in as a compass, directing them towards the supporting hug of iron-rich sustenance for ideal lung capability and in general prosperity.

Chapter 7

Harmonizing Nutrients
The Complete Ensemble

Fitting Supplements: The Total Gathering for Thorough Respiratory Wellbeing

In the perplexing coordination of respiratory wellbeing, an ensemble of supplements assumes an agreeable part, each note adding to the general essentialness of the lungs. This total outfit of supplements, painstakingly chose and adjusted, structures the foundation of a comprehensive way to deal with respiratory wellbeing. From cell reinforcements to omega-3 unsaturated fats, nutrients, and minerals, the excursion toward ideal lung capability envelops a different exhibit of dietary parts, each with its remarkable reverberation in supporting the perplexing dance of respiratory essentialness.

Cell reinforcement Hints: A Preface to Respiratory Protection

Cell reinforcements arise as the virtuosos in the gathering, making hints of safeguard against oxidative pressure - a central member in the domain of respiratory wellbeing. Nutrients C and E, alongside selenium and beta-carotene, stand as forefront protectors, killing free revolutionaries that might think twice about tissues.

The collaboration of these cell reinforcements frames a hearty safeguard, sustaining the respiratory framework against the oxidative difficulties presented by ecological toxins and the normal maturing process.

Omega-3 Unsaturated fats: The Melodic Progression of Respiratory Reverberation

The melodic progression of respiratory reverberation tracks down its mood in the omega-3 unsaturated fats, with docosahexaenoic corrosive (DHA) and eicosapentaenoic corrosive (EPA) becoming the dominant focal point. Found bounteously in greasy fish, for example, salmon, these fundamental unsaturated fats weave a story of calming ability. Their capacity to balance irritation gives a contrast to the provocative cycles that, when uncontrolled, may add to respiratory sicknesses. The omega-3 ensemble stretches out its range to bronchial wellbeing, advancing adaptability and versatility in the aviation routes.

Vitamin D: Sunlit Rhythm for Respiratory Strength

The sunlit rhythm of vitamin D resounds profoundly in the gathering, affecting respiratory strength with its multi-layered influence. Past its notable job in calcium retention for bone wellbeing, vitamin D shows immunomodulatory impacts, improving the respiratory resistant reaction. Satisfactory vitamin D levels have been connected to a decreased gamble of respiratory contaminations, and its lack might stir up misgivings about lung capability. The amicable transaction of daylight and vitamin D turns into an essential development in the ensemble of respiratory prosperity.

Magnesium: Cell Amicability and Oxygenation

As the director of cell congruity, magnesium organizes an orchestra inside the cells, adding to the ideal capability of chemicals engaged with energy creation and oxygen transport. The cadenced dance of magnesium inside mitochondria, the cell forces to be reckoned with, improves respiratory imperativeness by supporting ATP blend. Besides, magnesium's job in bronchodilation advances the unwinding of bronchial smooth muscles, working with the progression of air in the lungs.

Zinc: Cell Strength and Insusceptible Reverberation

Zinc arises as a robust individual from the outfit, assuming a double part in cell versatility and safe reverberation. Its association in the upkeep of cell films guarantees the underlying honesty of respiratory tissues. Additionally, zinc's immunomodulatory impacts add to the safeguard against respiratory diseases. The zinc-rich rhythm upholds the unpredictable equilibrium of invulnerable reactions, forestalling the disagreement that might prompt respiratory difficulties.

Vitamin A: Visionary Help for Mucosal Stronghold

In the vision of respiratory health, vitamin A takes on a job of visionary help, strengthening mucosal surfaces inside the respiratory lot. The mucosal linings go about as a defensive obstruction, and vitamin An assumes a significant part in keeping up with their respectability.

From the nasal entries to the bronchi, the vitamin A rhythm guarantees that the respiratory mucosa stays versatile against outer trespassers, adding to the first line of guard in quite a while.

Selenium: Cell Guardianship and Cancer prevention agent Congruity

Selenium takes on the position of cell guardianship inside the troupe, using its impact as a fundamental part of cancer prevention agent chemicals. These compounds, for example, glutathione peroxidase, go about as overseers, safeguarding cells from oxidative harm. Selenium's cancer prevention agent congruity reaches out to the respiratory framework, where it adds to the insurance of lung tissues against the attack of free revolutionaries. The selenium-rich hold back turns into an imperative part in the respiratory safeguard symphony.

L-ascorbic acid: Respiratory Rebuilding and Collagen Crescendo

In the crescendo of respiratory rebuilding, L-ascorbic acid starts to lead the pack, organizing the blend of collagen - a primary protein that bestows flexibility to lung tissues. Past its part in collagen arrangement, L-ascorbic acid displays cell reinforcement properties, killing free revolutionaries that might emerge during respiratory difficulties. The collagen crescendo turns into a foundation in keeping up with the flexibility and strength of the lungs, adding to their general capability.

Iron: Oxygen Transport Artful dance and Hemoglobin Concordance

In the artful dance of oxygen transport, iron plays out a smooth dance, working with the combination of hemoglobin - the iron-holding protein inside red platelets. This hemoglobin amicability is fundamental for the productive carriage of oxygen from the lungs to tissues all through the body. Iron's reverberation in respiratory health stretches out to the avoidance of lack of iron frailty, which, if neglected, may think twice about conveyance and add to respiratory weariness.

Vitamin K: Coagulation Rhythm and Lung Wellbeing

Vitamin K strides into the coagulation rhythm, impacting blood thickening and guaranteeing the uprightness of veins, including those inside the lungs. The amicable transaction of vitamin K with proteins engaged with coagulation adds to the counteraction of inordinate draining and upholds the microcirculation fundamental for lung wellbeing. The vitamin K development turns into a defensive musicality, protecting against likely vascular difficulties inside the respiratory framework.

Copper: Connective Tissue Intermingling and Respiratory Flexibility

Copper merges with connective tissues, assuming a vital part in the union of elastin - a protein that keeps up with the flexibility of lung tissues. This connective tissue intermingling guarantees the adaptability of aviation routes and supports lung capability.

Moreover, copper takes part in cancer prevention agent responses, improving the respiratory guard component. The copper-imbued reverberation turns into a watchman of respiratory strength, adding to the general essentialness of the lungs.

B Nutrients: Metabolic Ensemble and Energy Organization

The B nutrients combine efforts to make a metabolic ensemble, coordinating energy creation inside cells. B-complex nutrients, including B1 (thiamine), B2 (riboflavin), B3 (niacin), B5 (pantothenic corrosive), B6 (pyridoxine), B7 (biotin), B9 (folate), and B12 (cobalamin), assume fundamental parts in changing over supplements into energy. This energy arrangement is necessary to respiratory capability, supporting the requests of breathing and cell breath. The B nutrient orchestra turns into a unique development in the respiratory troupe.

Phytonutrients: Ensemble of Plant-Inferred Agreement

The ensemble of respiratory wellbeing reverberates with the consideration of phytonutrients - bioactive mixtures found in plant-based food sources. Flavonoids, carotenoids, and polyphenols, among others, add to the cell reinforcement and mitigating parts of the troupe. These plant-determined harmonies offer a range of advantages, from safe help to tweak of incendiary reactions, improving the respiratory orchestra with the dynamic shades of plant-based nourishment.

Orchestrating All encompassing Practices: The Closing Crescendo

In the closing crescendo of the total supplement gathering, recognizing the job of all encompassing practices in respiratory wellness is basic. Past individual supplements, the cooperative energy of a reasonable eating regimen, normal actual work, satisfactory hydration, and care establishes an amicable climate for ideal lung capability. All encompassing respiratory consideration stretches out to way of life decisions that limit openness to natural contaminations, advance respiratory cleanliness, and sustain by and large prosperity.

7.1 Synthesize the nutritional elements discussed in previous chapters

Orchestrating the Nourishing Embroidery: An Extensive Representation of Respiratory Health

In the embroidery of respiratory health, the orchestra of supplements examined in past sections winds around a thorough and mind boggling picture. Each nourishing component contributes an exceptional shade to the material, framing a comprehensive methodology that resounds with the imperativeness of the lungs. As we blend the different strings of cell reinforcements, omega-3 unsaturated fats, nutrients, minerals, and phytonutrients, a rich and amicable story arises, offering experiences into the exchange of nourishment and respiratory wellbeing.

Cancer prevention agents: Watchmen of Respiratory Trustworthiness

At the very front of the wholesome outfit, cell reinforcements arise as sturdy watchmen of respiratory honesty. Nutrients C and E, selenium, and beta-carotene structure a vigorous safeguard against oxidative pressure, killing free revolutionaries that could think twice about sensitive tissues of the lungs. This cell reinforcement ensemble expands its defensive reverberation, bracing the respiratory framework as well as going about as a safeguard against the natural attacks that describe present day living.

Omega-3 Unsaturated fats: The Mitigating Suggestion

The omega-3 unsaturated fats, DHA and EPA, play out a mitigating suggestion inside the nourishing ensemble. Found in overflow in greasy fish like salmon, these fundamental unsaturated fats regulate fiery cycles, offering a contradiction to the irritation that, when unrestrained, may add to respiratory difficulties. The omega-3 ensemble stretches out its impact to bronchial wellbeing, advancing adaptability and versatility in the aviation routes, guaranteeing the smooth progression of the respiratory tune.

Nutrients: A Multi-layered Melody for Respiratory Life

Nutrients stand as a multi-layered melody, each assuming a remarkable part in sustaining respiratory power. Vitamin D, with its sunlit rhythm, not just guides in that frame of mind for bone wellbeing yet additionally shows immunomodulatory impacts essential for respiratory resistant reactions. Vitamin A, a visionary help, sustains mucosal surfaces, going about as a forefront safeguard against outer trespassers in the respiratory plot. L-ascorbic acid arranges the combination of collagen, adding to the flexibility and strength of lung tissues, while vitamin K guarantees the coagulation rhythm that upholds vascular uprightness inside the lungs.

Minerals: Establishment Stones of Respiratory Strength

Inside the establishment stones of respiratory versatility, minerals become the overwhelming focus. Magnesium, with its cell congruity, works with energy creation and bronchodilation, upgrading the general essentialness of the respiratory framework. Zinc expects a double job in cell strength and safe reverberation, guaranteeing the underlying honesty of respiratory tissues and adding to guard against contaminations. Selenium, through its cell guardianship, shields lung tissues from oxidative harm, adding one more layer of safeguard to the respiratory outfit. Copper unites with connective tissues, supporting the amalgamation of elastin and keeping up with the adaptability of aviation routes.

Iron: The Expressive dance of Oxygen Transport and Hemoglobin Agreement

In the artful dance of oxygen transport, iron leads the dance, organizing the amalgamation of hemoglobin inside red platelets. This hemoglobin congruity is critical for the productive carriage of oxygen from the lungs to tissues all through the body. Iron's reverberation in respiratory health reaches out past oxygen transport, forestalling iron lack pallor, a condition that could think twice about conveyance and add to respiratory weariness.

The iron-rich expressive dance guarantees a consistent progression of oxygen, an essential development in the respiratory ensemble.

B Nutrients: A Unique Development in the Metabolic Ensemble

The B nutrients meet up in a powerful development, coordinating the metabolic ensemble that fills energy creation inside cells. Thiamine, riboflavin, niacin, pantothenic corrosive, pyridoxine, biotin, folate, and cobalamin by and large add to the change of supplements into energy, supporting the requests of breathing and cell breath. This energy organization frames a powerful development in the respiratory outfit, guaranteeing that the lungs have the fundamental fuel for their consistent and essential capability.

Phytonutrients: Dynamic Tones in the Plant-Determined Agreement

The ensemble of respiratory health resounds with the consideration of phytonutrients - dynamic tones in the plant-determined congruity. Flavonoids, carotenoids, and polyphenols add to the cancer prevention agent and calming parts of the troupe. These plant-inferred harmonies offer a range of advantages, from invulnerable help to the tweak of provocative reactions, enhancing the respiratory orchestra with the dynamic quality of plant-based nourishment. The phytonutrient rhythm turns into a fundamental note in the coordination of respiratory prosperity.

All encompassing Practices: The Closing Crescendo

In the closing crescendo, recognizing the job of all encompassing practices in respiratory wellness is essential. Past individual supplements, the collaboration of a fair eating regimen, normal actual work, satisfactory hydration, and care establishes an amicable climate for ideal lung capability. Comprehensive respiratory consideration reaches out to way of life decisions that limit openness to natural poisons, advance respiratory cleanliness, and support in general prosperity. The finishing up crescendo incorporates the aggregate of way of life factors that add to the continuous ensemble of respiratory imperativeness.

Embracing the Continuous Ensemble of Respiratory Essentialness

As we embrace the continuous ensemble of respiratory essentialness, the integrated representation uncovers a nuanced interaction among nourishment and lung well-being. The different components - cell reinforcements, omega-3 unsaturated fats, nutrients, minerals, phytonutrients, and all encompassing practices - combine into a thorough methodology that cultivates the flexibility and energy of the respiratory framework. As people set out on their excursion toward ideal lung capability, they become dynamic members in this orchestra, pursuing careful decisions that resound with the amicability of respiratory prosperity. The embroidery of respiratory well-being, woven with the strings of different supplements and all encompassing practices, remains as a demonstration of the many-sided and interconnected nature of sustaining the lungs for a long period of respiratory essentialness.

7.2 Create comprehensive meal plans for lung health

Ideal Sustenance for Respiratory Wellbeing: Complete Feast Plans

Making thorough feast plans for lung wellbeing includes choosing various supplement thick food sources that give fundamental nutrients, minerals, cell reinforcements, and different mixtures that help respiratory capability. These feast plans are intended to advance lung wellbeing, taking into account the mitigating, cell reinforcement, and wholesome angles essential for ideal respiratory health.

Feast Plan 1: Omega-3 Rich Joys

Breakfast: Salmon and Avocado Toast

Barbecued or heated salmon filet served on entire grain toast

Pounded avocado spread over the toast

Cut tomatoes and a sprinkle of chia seeds on top

A side of blended berries for added cell reinforcements

Lunch: Quinoa and Spinach Salad with Pecan Dressing

Quinoa base with new spinach leaves

Cherry tomatoes, cucumber, and red chime peppers for added nutrients

Barbecued chicken or tofu for protein

Thrown with a pecan based dressing for omega-3 unsaturated fats

Nibble: Greek Yogurt Parfait

Plain Greek yogurt layered with blueberries and strawberries

Shower with honey and sprinkle with squashed flaxseeds for extra supplements

Supper: Heated Cod with Yam Pound and Broccoli

Heated cod filets prepared with spices and lemon

Pounded yams for a portion of vitamin A

Steamed broccoli for added fiber and cancer prevention agents

Dinner Plan 2: Cell reinforcement Rich Joy

Breakfast: Berry and Spinach Smoothie Bowl

Mix together spinach, blended berries, banana, and a sprinkle of almond milk

Top with granola, cut almonds, and a sprinkle of honey for added surface

Lunch: Chickpea and Vegetable Sautéed food

Sautéed chickpeas with vivid ringer peppers, broccoli, and snap peas

Thrown with a light sesame-ginger sauce

Served over earthy colored rice for complex starches

Nibble: Avocado and Tomato Bruschetta

Cut cherry tomatoes and avocado on entire grain saltines

Sprinkle with basil and a smidgen of balsamic coating

Supper: Barbecued Chicken with Quinoa and Simmered Vegetables

Barbecued chicken bosom prepared with spices and lemon

Quinoa cooked with vegetable stock for added character

Broiled Brussels fledglings, carrots, and asparagus as an afterthought

Dinner Plan 3: Supplement Pressed Plant-Based Enjoyments

Breakfast: Green Smoothie with Nut Margarine Toast

Mix spinach, kale, banana, and almond milk for a green smoothie

Entire grain toast finished off with almond or peanut butter

Lunch: Lentil and Vegetable Soup

Generous lentil soup with carrots, celery, tomatoes, and kale

Sprinkle with nourishing yeast for added nutrients

Nibble: Hummus and Veggie Platter

Newly cut cucumber, carrot sticks, and ringer pepper cuts

Matched with hummus for a fantastic and nutritious bite

Supper: Broiled Vegetable Quinoa Bowl

Broiled yams, Brussels fledglings, and cauliflower

Served over a bed of quinoa

Showered with a tahini dressing for added character

Dinner Plan 4: Iron-Rich Blowout

Breakfast: Spinach and Feta Omelet

Whisked eggs collapsed with new spinach and feta cheddar

Presented with a side of entire grain toast

Lunch: Turkey and Kale Wrap

Entire grain wrap loaded up with lean turkey cuts, kale, and cut tomatoes

A dab of Greek yogurt or tzatziki for added richness

Nibble: Trail Blend in with Nuts and Seeds

A blend of almonds, pecans, pumpkin seeds, and dried berries

A small bunch gives a supplement rich tidbit

Supper: Meat and Vegetable Sautéed food with Earthy colored Rice

Pan-seared lean hamburger strips with vivid vegetables like broccoli, ringer peppers, and snap peas

Served over earthy colored rice for a healthy and fiber-rich feast

Key Contemplations for Lung-Quality Dinner Plans:

Hydration: Satisfactory water admission is urgent for in general wellbeing and respiratory capability. Incorporate water, home grown teas, and imbued water with cuts of citrus natural products or cucumber.

Segment Control: Focus on segment sizes to keep a solid weight, which is fundamental for lung wellbeing.

Assortment: Go for the gold of natural products, vegetables, entire grains, lean proteins, and sound fats to guarantee a different scope of supplements.

Limit Handled Food varieties: Limit the admission of handled and refined food sources, which might add to irritation and other medical problems.

Think about Dietary Limitations: Designer feast plans to individual dietary requirements, considering sensitivities, prejudices, or explicit medical issue.

Careful Eating: Practice careful eating by focusing on craving and completion signs. Bite food completely and enjoy each nibble.

Talk with an Expert: Prior to rolling out huge dietary improvements, particularly for people with previous medical issue, talk with a medical services proficient or an enlisted dietitian.

7.3 Encourage readers to adopt a balanced, nutrient-rich lifestyle for sustained respiratory well-being

Supporting Respiratory Prosperity: Embracing a Decent, Supplement Rich Way of life

In the orchestra of life, our respiratory wellbeing assumes an essential part, directing the cadence of our reality. Embracing a decent, supplement rich way of life isn't simply a decision; it is an amicable obligation to the supported prosperity of our lungs - the quiet orchestrators of each and every breath we take. As we set out on this excursion towards respiratory imperativeness, it's significant to comprehend the significant effect our way of life decisions can have on the perplexing orchestra of our respiratory framework.

Grasping the Significance of Respiratory Wellbeing:

Our lungs, as determined entertainers in an ensemble, energetically execute the undertaking of providing oxygen to each phone in our body. They explore the intricacies of our breath, giving life-supporting oxygen and ousting carbon dioxide. In any case, the requests put on our respiratory framework are elevated in our contemporary climate, overflowing with contamination, stationary ways of life, and dietary decisions that may not necessarily support ideal lung capability.

The meaning of respiratory health stretches out past the aversion of ailment; it impacts our general essentialness and personal satisfaction. Solid lungs add to expanded energy levels, worked on resistant capability, and an uplifted feeling of prosperity. Subsequently, cultivating respiratory wellbeing turns into a significant demonstration of taking care of oneself, a pledge to supporting the actual embodiment of life inside us.

The Supplement Rich Ensemble: A Way of life Song of devotion for Respiratory Imperativeness:

A fair, supplement rich way of life frames the song of devotion for supported respiratory prosperity. There's really no need to focus on intense changes or transitory fixes yet rather an agreeable combination of healthy practices into our day to day routines. We should investigate the key support points that create this way of life hymn, directing us towards the supported essentialness of our lungs.

1. **Healthy Sustenance:**

   At the core of respiratory health lies the fuel we give to our bodies. Choose a different, plant-driven diet wealthy in organic products, vegetables, entire grains, lean proteins, and solid fats. These food sources supply a plenty of nutrients, minerals, cell reinforcements, and phytonutrients, making an ensemble of sustenance for our lungs. Embrace the energetic shades of nature on your plate, for each tint brings a remarkable arrangement of supplements that adds to the general soundness of your respiratory framework.

   Consolidate omega-3 unsaturated fats, tracked down in greasy fish, flaxseeds, and pecans, for their mitigating properties that resound with the concordance of respiratory prosperity. Investigate the supplement rich suggestion of salad greens, which house a range of nutrients, including vitamin An and vitamin K critical for mucosal stronghold and coagulation support.

   Take part in the artful dance of oxygen transport with iron-rich food sources like lean meats, vegetables, and salad greens. These food sources work with the combination of hemoglobin, guaranteeing the consistent progression of oxygen from the lungs to each cell in the body. The supplement rich orchestra is a festival of culinary variety, an excursion where each chomp adds to the crescendo of respiratory imperativeness.

2. **Actual Concordance:**

   The stationary ways of life that portray current living can make a conflicting note in the orchestra of respiratory wellbeing. Active work, in its horde structures, is the way to reestablishing congruity. Whether through energetic strolls, strengthening runs, yoga, or dance, development upgrades lung limit, further develops flow, and supports by and large respiratory capability.

   Participate in exercises that advance profound, diaphragmatic breathing, for example, profound stomach breathing activities or pranayama. These practices fortify respiratory muscles as well as encourage a careful association with our breath, advancing a feeling of quiet and unwinding.

   Consider integrating obstruction preparing into your everyday practice to upgrade by and large muscle strength, incorporating the muscles associated with relaxing. A reasonable and normal activity routine turns into a development ensemble that blends with the many-sided dance of respiratory prosperity.

3. **Hydration Melody:**

Water is the remedy of life, and its part in respiratory wellbeing is frequently misjudged. Remaining satisfactorily hydrated guarantees the diminishing of bodily fluid in the aviation routes, working with its leeway and lessening the gamble of respiratory contaminations. Hydration additionally upholds the mucosal linings of the respiratory plot, adding to their honesty and strength.

Imbue your hydration routine with home grown teas, warm water with lemon, or implanted water with cuts of cucumber or mint. These options improve flavor as well as deal extra supplements and cell reinforcements, adding to the generally respiratory song.

4. **Supportive Rest:**

The nighttime break of rest is a crucial development in the orchestra of respiratory imperativeness. Quality rest upholds the body's maintenance instruments, including the recharging of respiratory tissues and the guideline of invulnerable capability. Go for the gold long periods of helpful rest every evening, making a nighttime ensemble that blends with the necessities of your respiratory framework.

Lay out a quieting pre-rest schedule, darkening lights, and keeping away from electronic gadgets basically an hour prior to sleep time. Make a rest safe-haven with an agreeable sleeping cushion and pads, permitting the nighttime ensemble to unfurl in a climate helpful for profound, peaceful sleep.

5. **Stress Tune:**

The effect of weight on respiratory wellbeing is a nuanced tune that requires cautious thought. Ongoing pressure can add to shallow breathing examples, compound respiratory circumstances, and compromise resistant capability. Incorporating pressure the executives methods, like care, contemplation, or profound breathing activities, turns into a melodic contradiction that reestablishes concordance to the respiratory ensemble.

Develop snapshots of quietness and reflection, permitting the pressure tune to change into a peaceful melody. Investigate rehearses that reverberate with your singular inclinations, whether it's tendency strolls, workmanship, music, or essentially snapshots of calm thought. Stress the executives turns into a fundamental development in the arrangement of supported respiratory prosperity.

6. **Ecological Amicability:**

Our outer climate fundamentally impacts the respiratory ensemble. Be aware of indoor air quality, limiting openness to contaminations, allergens, and aggravations. Guarantee legitimate ventilation in living spaces, think about air purifiers, and stay away from tobacco smoke.

Whenever the situation allows, invest energy in open air spaces with natural air and plant life. Nature itself offers an orchestra of respiratory advantages, from the oxygen-delivering limit of plants to the quieting impact of regular environmental factors.

7. **All encompassing Medical care Tune-Up:**

Ordinary medical services check-ups become the tuning fork that guarantees the continuous reverberation of respiratory wellbeing. Intermittent lung capability tests, screenings, and discussions with medical services experts help screen and address any expected issues. A preventive song considers early mediation and changes in the orchestra of respiratory consideration.

The Continuous Orchestra of Respiratory Essentialness:

Embracing a decent, supplement rich way of life is a challenge to take part in the continuous orchestra of respiratory essentialness. Every decision we make, from the food varieties we relish to the developments we take part in, adds to the amicable prosperity of our lungs. It's an orchestra where the rhythm of sustenance, actual work, hydration, rest, stress the executives, natural contemplations, and comprehensive medical care meets into a melodic embroidery of respiratory wellbeing.

As dynamic members in this ensemble, we hold the guide's implement, directing the developments with careful decisions and supporting practices. The continuous obligation to a fair, supplement rich way of life turns into a long lasting organization with our respiratory prosperity. It is a song of praise of taking care of oneself, a tune that resonates through the breaths we take, supporting the essentialness of our lungs for a long period of wellbeing and concordance. In this continuous ensemble, each note, every development, turns into a demonstration of our obligation to the supported prosperity of the quiet entertainers inside - our lungs.